Cardiovascular
Regulation

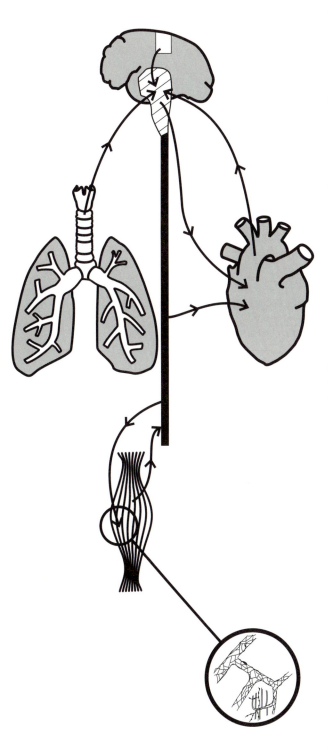

Cardiovascular Regulation

Editors
David Jordan
Janice Marshall

PORTLAND PRESS

Published by Portland Press, 59 Portland Place, London W1N 3AJ, U.K.
on behalf of the Physiological Society
In North America orders should be sent to Ashgate Publishing Co.,
Old Post Road, Brookfield, VT 05036-9704, U.S.A.

ISBN 1 85578 024 0   ISSN 0969-8116

British Library Cataloguing in Publication Data
A catalogue record for this book is available from
the British Library

Although, at the time of going to press, the information contained in this publication is believed to be correct, neither the authors nor the publisher assume any responsibility for any errors or omissions herein contained. Opinions expressed in this book are those of the authors and are not necessarily held by the editors or the publishers.

Cover illustration by T. Beer
Book design by A. Moyes

Typeset by Portland Press Ltd. and printed in Great Britain by the
University Press, Cambridge.

Contents

Preface   vii

Abbreviations   ix

1
**Central nervous integration of   1
cardiovascular regulation**
D. Jordan

2
**Aspects of the integration of the   15
respiratory and cardiovascular systems**
M. de Burgh Daly

3
**Cardiovascular changes associated   37
with behavioural alerting**
J.M. Marshall

4
**Cardiovascular changes   61
associated with sleep**
J.M. Marshall

5
Regulation of blood volume   77
R. Hainsworth and M.J. Drinkhill

6
**Cardiovascular responses to exercise: 93
central and reflex contribution**
J.H. Coote

7
**Metabolic control of blood flow   113
with reference to heart, skeletal
muscle and brain**
M.D. Brown

8
**Changing perspectives on   127
microvascular fluid exchange**
J.R. Levick

Glossary   153

Index   157

v

Preface

This book, the second in the series Studies in Physiology, arose out of presentations at a Physiological Society Teaching Symposium held at the Royal Free Hospital Medical School in February 1991. At that time we felt it was opportune to arrange such a symposium to inform Teachers of Physiology about the numerous changes that had taken place in current views on Control of the Circulation, especially since many of these were only slowly being taken up by the standard student textbooks. Subsequently, we felt that the ideas expressed at the symposium deserved a wider audience.

The text begins with an overview of the role of the central nervous system in regulating the cardiovascular system. This is followed by detailed descriptions of how the cardiovascular and respiratory systems interact during physiological situations, such as during stimulation of the arterial chemoreceptors, during diving, alerting and fear, when asleep or when exercising. In particular, for each situation there is discussion of how the central nervous system can either integrate individual reflex responses or evoke patterns of autonomic outflow appropriate for that situation. The control of intra- and extravascular fluid volumes — from the level of the whole body to the capillary — is then discussed in chapters on the regulation of blood volume, local control of blood flow to individual vascular beds and the regulation of fluid filtration across capillaries. We hope the book will be of interest to undergraduate students and their teachers: the summary boxes and review references cited as Essential Reading reflect this. In addition, for those stimulated to study the subject to a greater depth, each chapter also provides for Further Reading to cover the subject to postgraduate level.

David Jordan
Janice M. Marshall

Abbreviations

ANP	atrial natriuretic peptide
C_i	interstitial protein concentration
C_L	lymph protein concentration
C_p	plasma protein concentration
CSF	cerebrospinal fluid
CVLM	caudal ventrolateral medulla
CVM	cardiac vagal motoneurone
DLH	D-L-homocysteic acid
DVN	dorsal vagal nucleus
ECG	electrocardiogram
EDHF	endothelium-derived hyperpolarizing factor
EDRF	endothelium-derived relaxing factor
EEG	electroencephalogram
GABA	γ–aminobutyric acid
IML	intermediolateral cell column
J receptor	juxta pulmonary capillary receptor
LTF	lateral tegmental field
MVC	maximum voluntary conductance
NA	nucleus ambiguus
NMDA	N-methyl-D-aspartate
NO	nitric oxide
NTS	nucleus tractus solitarius
$PaCO_2$	partial pressure (arterial) of carbon dioxide
PG	prostaglandin
P_i	inorganic phosphate
PO_2	partial pressure (arterial) of oxygen
RVLM	rostral ventrolateral medulla
SIDS	sudden infant death syndrome
TPR	total peripheral resistance

CNS integration of cardiovascular regulation

David Jordan
Department of Physiology, Royal Free Hospital and University College Medical School, Rowland Hill Street, London NW3 2PF, U.K.

Introduction

At rest, individuals show a basal level of arterial blood pressure and heart rate which, although variable, are maintained around some 'set point'; however, if the spinal cord is transected at the cervical level, the arterial blood pressure falls to low levels. Nevertheless, if the subject is subsequently well-maintained, at least some recovery of the blood pressure occurs. Denervation of the heart alters the heart rate in a characteristic fashion depending on the species. In resting adult man, the predominant activity is in the inhibitory cardiac vagal fibres so that surgical denervation or pharmacological blockade of the vagal drive to the heart leads to an increase in heart rate (tachycardia). Alterations in various cardiovascular parameters are normally restrained by cardiovascular reflexes but, during various physiological situations, patterns of autonomic activity are evoked which over-ride these individual reflex mechanisms. When considering control of the cardiovascular system, it is necessary to produce a scheme which will account for all of these factors and enable us to list a number of questions that we must be able to answer adequately. What is the origin of the nervous tone which maintains the resting arterial blood pressure? What is the origin of the nervous activity modulating pacemaker activity in the heart? What central neural pathways are responsible for the reflex buffering of cardiovascular parameters? How can the central nervous system organize patterns of autonomic and somatic activity appropriate for the particular physiological situation?

The vasomotor centre

The original concept of a 'vasomotor centre' in the medulla oblongata (Fig. 1) comes from the transection experiments performed by Dittmar and colleagues in the late nineteenth century. To this day, almost all physiological textbooks show (in some form or other) Fig. 1, which is taken from the work of Alexander [1] and which provides a modern synthesis of that earlier work. While recording arterial blood pressure and inferior cardiac nerve activity, he combined controlled brainstem transections with localized electrical stimulation of parts of the brainstem and afferent nerves. He proposed that the medulla could be divided into two discrete 'centres', mediating pressor (sympathoexcitatory) and depressor (sympathoinhibitory) responses, respectively. He concluded that the rostral pressor and caudal depressor centres were distinct entities, each with its own spinal output, and that each was independently capable of tonic activity. In addition, all reflexes producing sympathoexcitation or sympathoinhibition were mediated by pathways which acted via these medullary 'centres'.

While this model explained much of the known experimental data, there are now numerous pieces of evidence which make this hypothesis untenable. First, there is an underlying assumption that each variable that can be measured in the periphery must have a separate brainstem region controlling it. Although this idea is not untenable in itself, it would seem strange to extend it to include arterial blood pressure which is itself a variable, dependent on at least two other cardiovascular variables — cardiac output and peripheral resistance. Secondly, there is the assumption that all regions of the brain from which changes in a particular variable can be evoked must be linked together as a 'centre'. Again, while in theory this could indeed be true, we know now for instance that there are direct descending pathways to sympathetic preganglionic neurones from regions as disparate as the caudal medulla, the A5 nucleus of the pons and the paraventricular nucleus of the hypothalamus

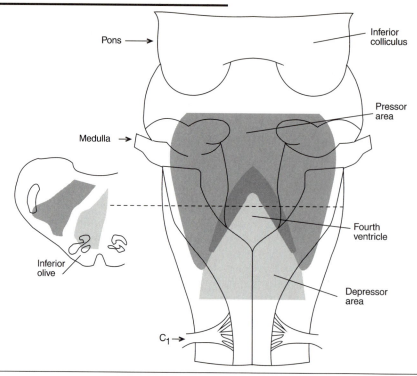

Fig. I. The dorsolateral pressor and ventromedial depressor regions projected onto the dorsal surface of the cat brainstem
On the left is shown a frontal section of the medulla at the level of the dashed line. Modified from [1].

[2,3] (Fig. 2). Electrical or chemical stimulation in each of these regions can modify sympathetic outflow independent of the other regions. Thirdly, we know now that the nucleus tractus solitarius (NTS), the site of termination of baroreceptor afferents, and the dorsal vagal nucleus (DVN) and nucleus ambiguus (NA), the location of vagal preganglionic neurones innervating the heart, are mainly within the defined 'pressor centre', even though activation of baroreceptor afferents will evoke a depressor response. Finally, on a semantic note, to define a region as a 'centre' implies an exclusivity which denies other functions for neurones within that region. Clearly, this cannot be the case and was probably not intended to be the implication. However, for this reason alone it would be better to abandon the term 'centre' in reference to both cardiovascular and to respiratory control. Indeed, we know now that the ongoing activity of some individual neurones in the brainstem reticular formation, which is within the 'vasomotor centre', can have rhythms related to cardiovascular inputs, the

respiratory cycle, somatosensory input and the electroencephalogram (EEG). Despite these major criticisms of the hypothesis, many authors of physiology textbooks seem unwilling to abandon the convenient Alexander model.

▶ The idea that cardiovascular regulation is effected via medullary 'vasomotor or cardiovascular centres' is no longer valid.
▶ We can now consider cardiovascular control as a series of individual reflexes which can act independently, can interact with one another or can be integrated into different patterns of response depending on the stimulus.

This vasomotor centre hypothesis has been used to describe both the origin of the tonic vasomotor activity and reflex control of the heart and blood vessels. If we are to disregard it, what can we put in its place to explain these two important facets of cardiovascular control?

The origin of vasomotor tone

There is now evidence in both resting animals and humans that blood vessels are normally in a state of partial constriction, and that this is due to ongoing activity in their sympathetic vasoconstrictor innervation [4,5]. When considering the origin of such vasoconstrictor activity, we need to deal with the control of activity in sympathetic nerves in general. This has recently been reviewed in detail [6,7]. Sympathetic preganglionic cell bodies are located in a column stretching the length of the thoracic and upper lumbar spinal cord. Within that portion of the neuraxis they are found, predominantly, within the intermediolateral cell column (IML) in the

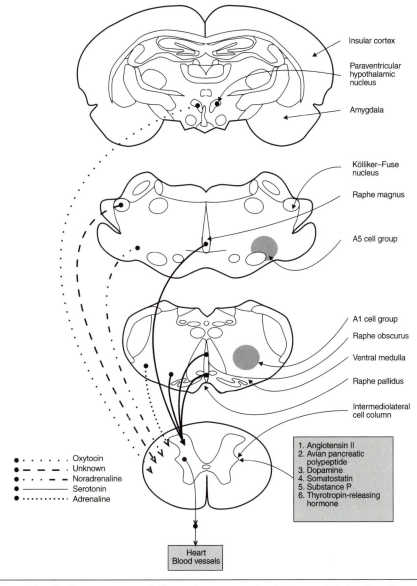

Fig. 2. **A summary of direct inputs to the intermediolateral cell column, the location of sympathetic preganglionic neurones**
Serotonergic inputs originate in raphe pallidus, raphe obscurus, raphe magnus and the ventral medulla. Noradrenaline- and adrenaline-containing neurones arise in the A5 and A1 cell groups, respectively. Adapted from [3] with permission.

lateral horn. A smaller group, sometimes termed the central autonomic nucleus, is found just dorsal and lateral to the central canal. In addition, scattered preganglionic neurones are found in the grey matter separating the central autonomic nucleus and the IML, and also extending into the white matter lateral to the IML. The axons of the majority of preganglionic neurones exit the spinal cord at the same segmental level, but a few will exit by spinal nerves one or two segments higher or lower down the spinal cord. This produces a rostro–caudal topographical organization of preganglionic neurones within the spinal cord, based on the level of segmental outflow. In addition, at each segmental level, there is some separation of neurones depending on their target nerve/organ and possibly on their function. This separation is far from absolute, and, on the basis of our knowledge so far, it is impossible to infer the function of a particular sympathetic preganglionic neurone based on its position within the spinal cord. In the near future, however, it may be possible to infer function from anatomical studies, since there is now a growing body of evidence from several groups that the neurochemical profile of both the neuronal cells and their inputs may be matched to their function.

Individual sympathetic preganglionic neurones receive synaptic information from a variety of sources. Spinal afferent inputs may arise directly from inputs at the same segmental level, or from inputs arriving at distant segments via intrinsic spinal interneurones. In addition, sympathetic preganglionic neuronal discharge is heavily influenced by activity in pathways descending in the ventral and lateral segments of the spinal cord from the brainstem and higher parts of the central nervous system [2,3]. In intact individuals, these descending inputs dominate the sympathetic outflow; however, after spinal section, the spinal sympathetic pathways can manifest themselves [6,7]. The descending pathways mediate both excitatory and inhibitory influences on sympathetic outflow, and it is believed that ongoing activity in one or more of the descending excitatory pathways is responsible for tonic activity in sympathetic outflow. These pathways originate in several sites in the brainstem (Fig. 2).

The following neurones have all been shown to project to the region of the IML [2,3]: catecholamine-containing neurones in the A5

region; serotonin-containing neurones in the caudal raphe nuclei (pallidus, magnus and obscurus) and in the B1 region lateral to raphe pallidus; neurones in the rostral ventrolateral medulla (RVLM; also known as nucleus paragigantocellularis lateralis) (see Chapter 3); in the dorsomedial NTS in the medulla; and Kölliker–Fuse nuclei of the pons. In addition, some oxytocin- and vasopressin-containing neurones in the paraventricular nucleus of the hypothalamus have been shown to have spinally projecting axons. However, the relative roles of these descending pathways have yet to be elucidated. It is possible that different pathways innervate different functional groups of sympathetic preganglionic neurones, or that different pathways are recruited during different physiological responses. This organization may underlie another important question of sympathetic function which has yet to be answered — where is the functional dedication of individual preganglionic neurones determined? The simple textbook view is that sympathetic outflow is a generalized system which acts as a single unit, but this is no longer tenable. In recordings from single pre- and postganglionic neurones, in both animals and humans, there is now ample evidence to show that sympathetic neurones with different functions respond differentially to certain stimuli. For example, vasomotor and sudomotor neurones innervating the same hindlimb respond differently to a baroreceptor stimulus, whereas vasomotor neurones innervating vasculature in the hind- and forelimb would act in the same manner [4].

Evidence is now accumulating that one particular group of 'presympathetic' neurones — those located in the RVLM — is of particular importance in cardiovascular control [8] (see also Chapter 3). This derived from a demonstration by Feldberg and colleagues that blood pressure fell dramatically when pentobarbitone, or the inhibitory amino acid glycine, was placed on a restricted region of the ventral medullary surface. Electrical or chemical lesions of this 'glycine-sensitive area' reduce arterial pressure to levels not dissimilar to those produced by spinal transection. Neurones have now been identified within the brain just below the surface of the glycine-sensitive area. These neurones have many of the properties expected of a neurone mediating excitatory inputs to vasomotor sympathetic preganglionic neurones:

they have axons which project to the regions of the spinal cord containing sympathetic preganglionic neurones, and their basal discharge rate is related to mean arterial blood pressure in the same way as lumbar sympathetic nerve discharge [8] (Fig. 3). This basal firing exhibits a marked pulse- and respiratory-related pattern, which is imposed by inputs from the arterial baroreceptors and central respiratory neurones, respectively, and which mirrors that seen in pre- and postganglionic sympathetic vasomotor neurones [6]. Many cardiovascular reflexes are thought to act via this region. Stimulation of arterial baroreceptors inhibits these neurones powerfully [8], while stimulation of the arterial chemoreceptors and small-diameter sciatic nerve afferents excites them. The reticulo-spinal neurones found in the RVLM are not a homogenous group; they can be differentiated into different groups on the basis of conduction velocity of their descending axons, the trans-

mitters they contain (a major group are the C1 adrenaline-containing neurones) and on their putative function. However, at present, the evidence seems to indicate that the group of baroreceptor-sensitive RVLM neurones and those containing adrenaline are not one and the same [9]. By microstimulating small groups of these neurones with excitant amino acids it appears that the RVLM region is composed of distinct but overlapping pools of presympathetic neurones (Fig. 4) with different functions [10]. These pools appear to be arranged topographically, on the basis of their functional effects rather than the region of the body they innervate. For example, microstimuli can evoke parallel changes in both hind- and forelimb vascular resistances, while renal sympathetic nerve activity is activated from a different site.

If the RVLM neurones are indeed providing the major source of excitatory input to sympathetic preganglionic neurones (and, there-

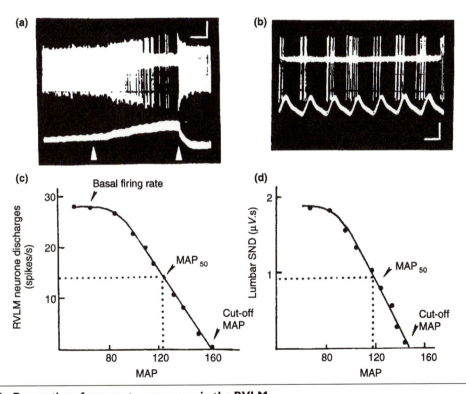

Fig. 3. **Properties of vasomotor neurones in the RVLM**

(a) Inhibition of neuronal discharges (upper trace) during a rise in arterial pressure (lower trace) evoked by restricting flow through the descending aorta. (b) On a faster timescale, the activity of the neurone is clearly related to the pulsatile activity in the arterial pressure wave.

(c) Relationship of mean discharge of the RVLM neurone and mean arterial pressure (MAP). (d) The lumbar sympathetic nerve discharge (SND) in the same preparation exhibits the same relationship with MAP. Reproduced with permission from [8].

fore, of vasomotor tone), then an important question is how do these neurones derive their ongoing activity? Stimulation within the 'defence areas' of the fore- or midbrain excites RVLM neurones (Fig. 4) (see also Chapter 3), and chemical or electrical lesions of the RVLM abolish the cardiovascular responses to defence area stimulation [10]. Thus it was proposed that tonic activation of the defence areas would provide the basis of tonic activity within neurones of the RVLM. This view simply pushes the vasomotor neurones back one stage, and the question then arises as to how these areas generate their activity. While they may indeed

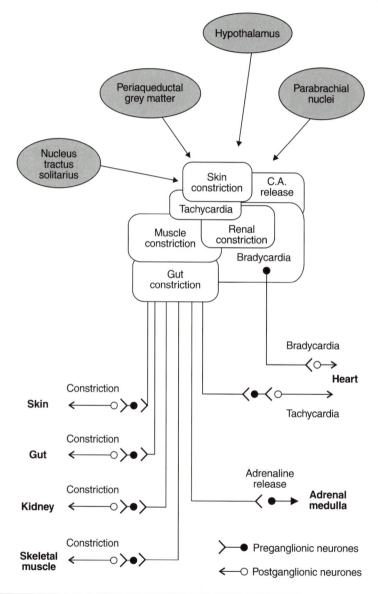

Fig. 4. Schematic diagram illustrating the connections and topographical organization of presympathetic neurones in the region of the RVLM

Distinct but overlapping neuronal pools within this area control the level of activity of sympathetic preganglionic neurones, which, in turn, modify the activity of pools of postganglionic fibres of specific function. Adapted from [10] with permission.

provide some of the ongoing drive in RVLM neurones, it has recently been suggested that some vasomotor RVLM neurones can exhibit intrinsic pacemaker activity [8]. When excitatory inputs to these neurones are blocked chemically, or reduced by inducing hypotension, then some of the cells adopt a regular, pacemaker-like discharge [8,9]. The cells showing pacemaker-like activity are not the C1 adrenaline-containing group of neurones which make up some 50% of the reticulo-spinal neurones in this region (Fig. 5). Although it has been demonstrated that under certain conditions some cells can show pacemaker activity, this is not proof that they themselves generate the vasomotor tone in the intact animal when they are in possession of their normal inputs. In this situation, their resting discharge will be modified by inputs from a variety of sources — arterial baroreceptor input will reduce their activity, while chemoreceptor drive and inputs from the hypothalamic defence area and periaqueductal grey will all increase it (Fig. 4).

An important role for RVLM neurones in controlling sympathetic outflow has now been proposed; however, it is important to remember that there are other pathways descending to the IML that may also have regulatory roles. If these other groups are investigated as thoroughly as the RVLM neurones, then a role for these may also be discovered. Indeed, Gebber and colleagues [11] have studied neurones in the lateral tegmental fields of the medulla. Some of these neurones are thought to be sympathoexcitatory, while others are thought to be sympathoinhibitory. Neither group has spinally projecting axons. Using the technique of spike-triggered averaging, Gebber proposed that the sympathoexcitatory neurones exert their influence by activating the RVLM sympathoexcitatory neurones described above; the sympathoinhibitory neurones exert their effects via caudal raphe–spinal neurones, independent of activity within the RVLM (Fig. 5). It is now clear that the brainstem contains the circuitry to generate a certain level of sympathetic tone. However, this does not exclude other levels of the neuraxis as also having an effect. Indeed, after high spinal section, the spinal cord itself can generate a certain level of sympathetic activity. In addition, after decerebration, sympathetic activity is reduced, suggesting that the

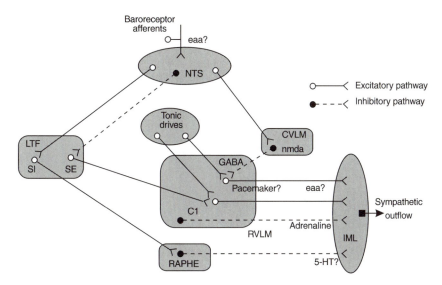

Fig. 5. Diagrammatic representation of the pathways by which activation of the arterial baroreceptors evokes inhibition of sympathetic vasoconstrictor nerve activity

Abbreviations used: C1, adrenaline-containing group of neurones; eaa, excitatory amino acid; LTF, lateral tegmental field; nmda, N-methyl-D-aspartate receptor; SE, sympathoexcitatory; SI, sympathoinhibitory; 5-HT, 5-hydroxytryptamine. Based on evidence in [2,8,11,17,19,20].

hypothalamus and/or forebrain regions also contribute to the resting level of vasomotor tone.

> ▶ Resting arterial blood pressure depends on a resting level of activity in the sympathetic vasoconstrictor outflow innervating blood vessels.
> ▶ This sympathetic nerve activity is the sum of both excitatory and inhibitory influences arising from a variety of sensory inputs and activity in various brain regions.
> ▶ A group of brainstem neurones in the RVLM is thought to provide tonic drive to the sympathetic outflow. This may arise from inherent pacemaker activity in these neurones.
> ▶ Sympathetic outflow is not controlled in a widespread manner as previously believed. There is differential control of sympathetic outflows based on their function.

Nervous control of the heart

Pacemaker cells in the sino-atrial node set a basal heart rate characteristic of the species. This tissue receives an innervation from both sympathetic and parasympathetic nerves. The prevailing level of heart rate at any instant is set by the balance of activities in these two innerva-tions, along with the effects of any circulating catecholamines, acting on the basal rhythm. In humans and dogs at rest, it is the vagal inhibitory innervation that predominates, but this varies from species to species. In addition, anaesthesia can differentially modify autonomic outflow so that what is characteristic of the anaesthetized animal is not always true in the awake state. In particular, anaesthesia tends to cause a rise in heart rate which can be explained by the observation that cardiac vagal outflow is depressed by a variety of anaesthetics [12].

Anatomical studies using retrograde tracing techniques now agree that vagal preganglionic neurones innervating the heart are found within two nuclei in the brainstem — the DVN and the NA [13]. Application of tracer substances, such as horseradish peroxidase or its conjugates, onto the individual intrathoracic cardiac branches of the vagus, or within the cardiac muscle itself, has demonstrated retrogradely labelled neurones in both these nuclei, with a few in an intermediate band of tissue between them (Fig. 6). However, the relative importance of the two nuclei seems to vary from species to species [14].

Anatomical studies can delineate the cells of origin of axons innervating heart tissue; however, unless the neurones are homogeneous, little can be deduced regarding the function of the visualized cells. Electrophysiological

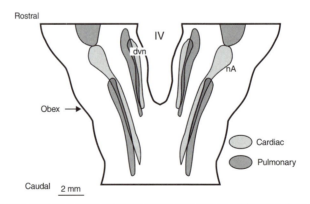

Fig. 6. Diagrammatic representation of the location within the brainstem of vagal preganglionic neurones innervating the heart and lungs

Preganglionic neurones are found in both the DVN and the NA. Although there is overlap, the pools of motoneurones innervating the heart and lungs are found in topographically distinct regions of the NA. Abbreviations used: dvn, dorsal vagal nucleus; nA, nucleus ambiguus; IV, fourth ventricle.

recordings of the activity of such neurones can help with this. While vagal motoneurones with axons projecting to the heart can be recorded in both of the vagal nuclei, neurones having properties consistent with a cardioinhibitory function are found almost exclusively within the NA of cats [15], but in both the NA and DVN of rabbits and rats [12,15]. Recordings from presumed cardioinhibitory neurones show that their ongoing activity is dependent, at least in part, upon the excitatory input they receive from the arterial baroreceptors. In addition, the arterial partial pressure of CO_2 ($PaCO_2$), acting via chemoreceptor inputs, can also provide a proportion of the basal vagal tone, since reduction of $PaCO_2$ by hyperventilation evokes tachycardia. Many other reflex inputs can also modify cardiac vagal outflow [12,16] (Fig. 7). In particular, inputs from pulmonary receptors and the central respiratory drive can markedly affect the level of vagal drive (see also Chapter 2). Vagal activity is reduced, leading to a rise in heart rate, both during the inspiratory phase of respiration, and when slowly adapting lung-stretch receptors are activated by lung inflation. Of course, under normal circumstances, both these effects would occur simultaneously and

this would explain the phenomenon of respiratory sinus arrhythmia, whereby heart rate increases during each inspiratory effort. Indeed, the degree of sinus arrhythmia is sometimes taken as an indicator of the level of vagal tone at any particular instance. Other airway receptors also have marked effects on the heart when activated; those in the upper airway and nasal passages evoke marked bradycardia as part of the 'diving response', while pulmonary and bronchial C-fibre afferents also excite vagal drive to the heart when stimulated. The question remains unanswered as to the function of those cardiac vagal motoneurones which do not have the properties assigned to cardioinhibitory neurones. In the cat, it has been proposed that there is an anatomical organization of vagal motoneurones — those in the NA being cardioinhibitory, while those in the DVN control ventricular contractility. However, although this idea is appealing, it has not been substantiated by subsequent experimental work. There is no information regarding the vagal preganglionic neurones which modify conduction through the atria-ventricular node, nor on the central organization of the parasympathetic innervation of coronary blood vessels, although

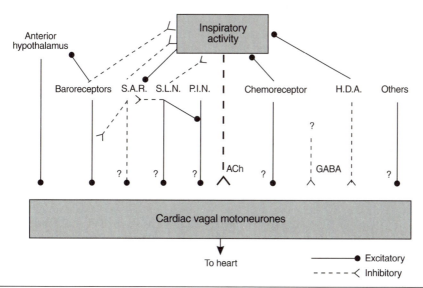

Fig. 7. **A summary of the possible mechanisms that interact at the level of the cardiac vagal motoneurones to evoke cardiac slowing**

Excitatory mechanisms are shown as solid lines, inhibitory mechanisms as dotted lines. The lines indicate pathways of unknown synaptic complexity, not individual neurones. Abbreviations used: ACh, acetylcholine; H.D.A., hypothalamic defence area; P.I.N., subpopulation of post-inspira- *tory neurones; S.A.R., slowly adapting, lung-stretch receptor afferents; S.L.N., superior laryngeal nerve afferents; ?, postulated pathways. Adapted with permission from [12].*

it is now accepted that certain reflex-evoked increases in coronary blood flow are mediated by such parasympathetic innervation.

▶ Parasympathetic preganglionic neurones innervating the heart are found in two vagal motor nuclei — the NA and the DVN.
▶ The tonic level of activity in this cardioinhibitory outflow is dependent on the excitatory inputs the neurones receive, including the arterial baroreceptors and chemoreceptors. In addition, these neurones are a site of integration for the many reflex inputs which alter heart rate.

Neural substrates mediating cardiovascular reflexes

Cranial sensory afferents arising from visceral structures terminate in the brainstem homologue of the dorsal horn, the NTS. This longitudinal nucleus in the dorsomedial medulla oblongata receives afferent information from all glossopharyngeal and vagal nerve afferents. In addition to gustatory afferents, these will include sensory afferents from the arterial baroreceptors and chemoreceptors, cardiac receptors, upper and lower airway and pulmonary receptors. The termination of the IXth nerve afferents is restricted to the rostral two-thirds of the nucleus, while the vagal afferents terminate in the caudal two-thirds. The intermediate part of the nucleus, which receives information from both vagal and glossopharyngeal afferents, is thought to be the most important region in terms of cardiovascular control (see Fig. 2 in Chapter 2). Considering data from both histological and neurophysiological studies, it is now clear that functionally different afferents terminate in different regions of the nucleus, though some overlap does occur [16,17] (Fig. 8). Baroreceptor afferents arising from either the aortic arch or carotid sinus project to similar regions of the NTS, predominantly the dorsal regions of the lateral and medial subnuclei on the ipsilateral side, with less-dense projections caudally to the medial and commissural subnuclei. In contrast, carotid chemoreceptor afferents terminate mainly in the dorsomedial, medial and commissural subnuclei of the NTS.

Receptor type	Divisions of the NTS		
	Medial	Commissural	Lateral
Myelinated aortic baroreceptor	● ● / ● ○	●	● ● / ● ●
Myelinated carotid baroreceptor	●	●	● ● ● / ● ● ●
Unmyelinated carotid baroreceptor	● ● / ●	●	● ● / ● ●
Unmyelinated carotid chemoreceptor	● ● ● ○ / ● ● ●	● ● ● ○ / ● ● ○	● ●
Myelinated lung SAR	● ● ● / ● ● ●		● ●
Myelinated lung RAR	● ● ○ / ● ● ○ ○	● ● ● ○ / ● ● ○ ○	● ●
Unmyelinated bronchial receptor	● ● ● ○ / ● ● ●	● ● ● ○ / ● ● ○	
Unmyelinated pulmonary receptor	● ● ● ○ / ● ●	● ● ● ○ / ● ●	

Fig. 8. **Summary of the major regions of termination within the NTS of the cat of cardiovascular and pulmonary afferents as determined by antidromic mapping studies [17]**
The relative density of ipsilateral (●) and contralateral (○) regions of termination is denoted by the number of dots; the most extensive regions of termination are shaded.

The main termination of slowly adapting pulmonary-stretch receptors is the medial subnucleus, with a less-dense projection to the lateral and ventrolateral subnuclei (the location of the 'dorsal respiratory group'). Indeed, one subgroup of the inspiratory neurones found here, the Iβ neurones, receives a monosynaptic excitatory input from such slowly adapting lung-stretch afferents. This input is distinct from the terminations of rapidly adapting pulmonary afferents, which are located more caudally in the NTS, in the medial and commissural subnuclei. Bronchial C-fibre afferents have a more extensive central termination than pulmonary C-fibre afferents, but their sites of projection are very similar. Both groups project mainly to the medial and commissural regions of the NTS and, unlike their myelinated counterparts, have little, if any, direct input to the lateral, ventrolateral or ventral subnuclei. Although limited, the amount of overlap of terminal fields, and the convergence of different afferent inputs onto postsynaptic neurones, is the neural substrate needed to give this nucleus a truly integrative function (Fig. 8).

Pathways from the NTS to the nuclei containing vagal preganglionic neurones and presympathetic bulbospinal neurones are now being elucidated. Using anatomical tracing methods, it has recently been demonstrated that NTS neurones can make monosynaptic connections with vagal motoneurones in the NA and the DVN, and with neurones in the ventrolateral regions of the medulla oblongata. However, these are probably few in number compared with the numerous multisynaptic pathways linking these different nuclei [18]. In addition, the latency between stimulation of afferent nerves and responses in vagal outflow is generally longer than would be expected if a simple monosynaptic connection between the NTS and the motoneurones was the prevalent pathway. No evidence is available as to the relative importance of the different reflex paths.

As described earlier, baroreceptor inhibition of sympathetic activity is probably mediated via inhibition of excitatory bulbospinal neurones in the RVLM, since the activity of spinally projecting RVLM neurones is reduced when blood pressure is raised. This inhibitory action is mediated by two or more separate brainstem pathways. The suppression of RVLM neurone activity is due to an inhibitory input mediated both by inhibitory postsynaptic potentials and via disfacilitation of an excitatory input [9] (Fig. 6). As yet, there is no direct evidence as to which of the excitatory pathways acting on RVLM neurones are inhibited by baroreceptor stimulation. However, sympathoexcitatory neurones in the lateral tegmental field excite RVLM neurones and are inhibited by baroreceptor stimulation [11]. The inhibitory pathway from the NTS to the RVLM is also indirect, uses γ-aminobutyric acid (GABA) as its neurotransmitter and acts via a group of neurones in the caudal ventrolateral medulla (CVLM) [19,20]. The CVLM includes the A1 group of catecholamine-containing neurones, but these are not thought to play a part in the baroreceptor-mediated decrease in sympathetic nerve activity. The baroreceptor pathway from the NTS excites CVLM neurones by releasing an excitatory amino acid which acts on N-methyl-D-aspartate (NMDA) receptors in the CVLM [19]. Inhibition of neurones in the CVLM by application of NMDA antagonists abolishes the depressor responses evoked by baroreceptor stimulation [19] and raises arterial blood pressure. Conversely, stimulation of CVLM neurones reduces blood pressure. The responses mediated by the CVLM require the integrity of the RVLM, since they are abolished

by disruption of activity in RVLM neurones [20]. Baroreceptor activation also excites sympathoinhibitory neurones in the lateral tegmental field. However, this effect on sympathetic outflow is independent of the RVLM, acting via descending inhibitory pathways originating in the raphe nuclei [11] (Fig. 2) (see also Chapter 4).

In addition to baroreceptor reflexes, there is now evidence that several other reflex alterations in vascular tone are blocked or attenuated when RVLM neurones are inhibited or chemically destroyed. These include the sympathoexcitatory responses evoked by stimulation of the cerebellar fastigial nucleus or somatic afferents in the sural and sciatic nerves.

While a purely brainstem network can be devised to explain individual reflex pathways, it is clear that other regions of the central nervous system can also be involved. For example, activation of arterial baroreceptors can excite neurones — not only in the medulla oblongata, but also in the parabrachial nucleus of the pons, in a variety of hypothalamic nuclei, in the amygdaloid nuclei and in the insular cortex [15,16]. Stimulation in the central nucleus of the amygdala in rabbits, or the anterior hypothalamus in cats, both of which receive baroreceptor information, leads to falls in heart rate, blood pressure, respiration and hindlimb vascular resistance. This pattern of response mirrors that evoked by raising carotid sinus pressure. In addition, lesions of the anterior hypothalamus attenuate the reflex responses caused by natural stimulation of the arterial baroreceptors [15]. Clearly then, parts of the neuraxis, in addition to the brainstem, may also be components of cardiovascular reflex pathways. Indeed, it is possible to conceive that these pathways form a longitudinal continuum throughout the neuraxis (Fig. 9). Many of the nuclei receiving cardiovascular afferent information, from which cardiovascular responses can be evoked, seem to show reciprocal connections. Hence, at each neural level, inputs arising from the periphery can integrate with others ascending and descending the neuraxis. The question then arises as to the role of these other regions. It would not seem unreasonable to suggest that simple brainstem or brainstem–spinal cord reflexes may operate during second-to-second homeostasis, while the other areas of the neuraxis can modulate or integrate these individual reflex responses into patterns of autonomic outflow relevant to the prevailing environmental situation.

Indeed, it is now known that the efficacy of many homeostatic reflexes is not fixed but can alter depending on the particular physiological situation. For example, as will be discussed in Chapter 2, the ability of arterial chemoreceptors to slow the heart and augment respiration is modified by the prevailing level of respiratory drive and by inputs from the face and nasal cavity (see Fig. 5 in Chapter 2) [16]. In addition, the gain and/or set point of the arterial baroreceptor reflex is modified during stress or the alerting reaction (see Chapter 3), in the different sleep states (see Chapter 4) and during muscular exercise (see Chapter 6) [16]. The sites at which such modulation occurs within the nervous system are various [15], but the NTS is one important site. During activation of the hypothalamic defence areas, chemoreceptor-sensitive neurones in the NTS receive excitatory inputs, whereas baroreceptor-sensitive neurones are inhibited by a chloride-dependent, inhibitory postsynaptic potential. This inhibition is mediated by the inhibitory transmitter GABA, which is probably released from local GABA-containing interneurones. In addition, these same baroreceptor-sensitive neurones can be inhibited by a GABA-mediated mechanism during activation of high-threshold muscle afferents or muscular contraction. Whether the same inhibitory pathways subserve both effects is not yet known. The inhibitory effect of hypothalamic defence-area stimulation on the baroreceptor reflex is also, in part, mediated at the level of the cardiac vagal motoneurones. It is at this site that the effects of central respiratory drive on cardiac reflexes are imposed [12]. The tachycardic effects of the defence response are probably due to both direct inhibitory effects on the cardiac vagal motoneurones and indirect effects due to augmentation of the inspiratory drive (see Fig. 4 in Chapter 2)

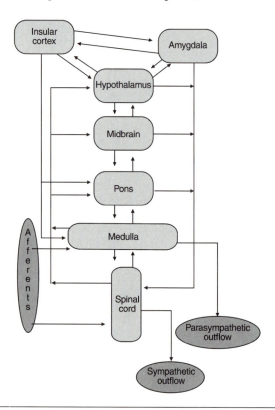

Fig. 9. **Schematic diagram of the possible interconnections between regions of the central nervous system now known to be involved in the central nervous integration of cardiovascular control [2,15, 16,18,21]**

▶ 'Cardiovascular' sensory afferent fibres terminate in the dorsal part of the medulla oblongata — in the NTS. Their terminations are, in part, organized topographically on the basis of the function of the receptor.

▶ NTS neurones relay to the presympathetic neurones in the RVLM and the cardiac vagal motoneurones by multisynaptic pathways. This is the basic organization of medullary–spinal reflexes.

▶ NTS neurones also project to 'higher' brain regions, where they can be integrated into more complex patterns of autonomic, behavioural and endocrine response.

▶ The efficacy of homeostatic reflexes is not constant but varies depending on the physiological situation. Many of these effects are imposed at the level of the NTS or the vagal cardiomotor neurones.

Patterns of autonomic and somatic behaviour

In normal physiological situations, we rarely measure individual reflex responses. It is much more usual for more than one reflex to be evoked at any particular instance. When this occurs we do not usually obtain a simple algebraic summation of the responses (see Chapter 2). Although homeostasis may rely on reflex alterations of cardiovascular parameters, it appears that the higher parts of the central nervous system are organized in such a way that, when activated, they evoke changes not in single variables but integrated patterns of autonomic, endocrine and somatic outflow; different independent variables combine to produce unique patterns of response according to the external stimulus evoking them. The longitudinal organization of the baroreceptor pathway discussed above can also be invoked for the integration of both the defence/alerting pattern of response [21] (see Chapter 3) and the pattern of cardiorespiratory outflow evoked during exercise (see Chapter 6). While teachers of physiology usually discuss skeletal motor control in terms of basic spinal reflexes, which are modified by pyramidal and extrapyramidal systems, programmed movements and so on, there is really no reason not to consider control of autonomic outflow in the same manner.

The author is grateful for the financial support of the Medical Research Council and Wellcome Trust which supported his research during the preparation of this review.

References

References [6,8,12,15–17] are essential reading.

1. Alexander, R.S. (1946) Tonic and reflex functions of medullary sympathetic cardiovascular centres. J. Neurophysiol. 9, 205–217
2. Loewy, A.D. (1990) Central autonomic pathways. In Central Regulation of Autonomic Functions (Loewy, A.D. and Spyer, K.M., eds.), pp. 88–103, Oxford University Press, Oxford
3. Loewy, A.D. and Neil, J.J. (1981) The role of descending monoaminergic systems in central control of blood pressure. Fed. Proc. 40, 2778–2785
4. Janig, W. (1985) Organization of the lumbar sympathetic outflow to skeletal muscle and skin of the cat hindlimb. Rev. Physiol. Biochem. Pharmacol. 102, 119–213
5. Wallin, B.G. and Fagius, J. (1988) Peripheral sympathetic neural activity in conscious humans. Annu. Rev. Physiol. 50, 565–576
6. Coote, J.H. (1988) The organisation of cardiovascular neurons in the spinal cord. Rev. Physiol. Biochem. Pharmacol. 110, 147–285
7. Laskey, W. and Polosa, C. (1988) Characteristics of the sympathetic preganglionic neuron and its synaptic input. Prog. Neurobiol. 31, 47–84
8. Guyenet, P.G. (1990) Role of the ventral medulla oblongata in blood pressure regulation. In Central Regulation of Autonomic Functions (Loewy, A.D. and Spyer, K.M., eds.), pp. 145–167, Oxford University Press, Oxford
9. Granata, A.R. and Kitai, S.T. (1992) Intracellular analysis *in vivo* of different barosensitive bulbospinal neurons in the rat ventrolateral medulla. J. Neurosci. 12, 1–20
10. Lovick, T.A. (1987) Cardiovascular control from neurones in the ventrolateral medulla. In Neurobiology of the Cardiorespiratory System (Taylor, E.W., ed.), pp. 197–208, Manchester University Press, Manchester
11. Gebber, G.L. (1990) Central determinants of sympathetic nerve discharge. In Central Regulation of Autonomic Functions (Loewy, A.D. and Spyer, K.M., eds.), pp. 126–144, Oxford University Press, Oxford
12. Jordan, D. and Spyer, K.M. (1987) Central neural mechanisms mediating respiratory–cardiovascular interactions. In Neurobiology of the Cardiorespiratory System (Taylor, E.W., ed.), pp. 322–341, Manchester University Press, Manchester
13. Hopkins, D.A. (1987) The dorsal motor nucleus of the vagus nerve and the nucleus ambiguus: structure and connections. In Cardiogenic Reflexes (Hainsworth, R., McWilliam, P.N. and Mary, D.A.S.G., eds.), pp. 185–203, Oxford University Press, Oxford
14. Withington-Wray, D.J., Taylor, E.W. and Metcalfe, J.D. (1987) The location and distribution of vagal preganglionic neurones in the hindbrain of lower vertebrates. In Neurobiology of the Cardiorespiratory System (Taylor, E.W., ed.), pp. 304–321, Manchester University Press, Manchester
15. Spyer, K.M. (1981) Neural organisation and control of the baroreceptor reflex. Rev. Physiol. Biochem. Pharmacol. 88, 23–124
16. Coleridge, H.M., Coleridge, J.C.G. and Jordan, D. (1991) Integration of ventilatory and cardiovascular control

systems. In The Lung: Scientific Foundations (Crystal, R.G. and West, J.B., eds.), pp. 1405–1418, Raven Press, New York

17. Jordan, D. and Spyer, K.M. (1986) Brainstem integration of cardiovascular and pulmonary afferent activity. Prog. Brain Res. **67**, 295–314

18. Luiten, P.G.M., ter Horst, G.J. and Steffans, A.B. (1987) The hypothalamus, intrinsic connections and outflow pathways to the endocrine system in relation to the control of feeding and metabolism. Prog. Neurobiol. **28**, 1–54

19. Gordon, F.J. (1987) Aortic baroreceptor reflexes are mediated by NMDA receptors in caudal ventrolateral medulla. Am. J. Physiol. **252**, R628–R633

20. Blessing, W.W. (1991) Inhibitory vasomotor neurons in the caudal ventrolateral medulla oblongata. News Physiol. Sci. **6**, 139–141

21. Jordan, D. (1990) Autonomic changes in affective behavior. In Central Regulation of Autonomic Functions (Loewy, A.D. and Spyer, K.M., eds.), pp. 349–366, Oxford University Press, Oxford

2

Aspects of the integration of the respiratory and cardiovascular systems

M. de Burgh Daly

Department of Physiology, Royal Free Hospital and University College School of Medicine, Rowland Hill Street, London NW3 2PF, U.K.

Interactions of the respiratory and cardiovascular systems

Respiration is controlled to maintain the correct arterial blood gas partial pressures (PaO_2 and $PaCO_2$) and pH, whereas the circulatory system is responsible for the transport of these gases to and from tissues. Thus, in any physiological situation, the respiratory and cardiovascular systems must act in concert: first to maintain constant, or as near constant as possible, the arterial blood gases and pH, and, secondly, to ensure that the metabolic needs of the tissues are met according to their demands for oxygen. It is evident that the control of respiration and the circulation cannot be independent of each other but must be integrated in such a way as to meet these criteria. The purpose of this review is, therefore, to examine some of the integrative mechanisms that operate between the two systems.

In naturally occurring situations affecting the cardiovascular system there is rarely, if ever, a change in activity of one input to the nervous system without others being affected at the same time. So that by central integration, the pattern of cardiovascular response evoked by each input is modified by other inputs causing the observed responses that are obtained in a particular situation (Fig. 1). Although we now have considerable knowledge of the pattern of response elicited by excitation of individual cardiovascular receptor groups, there is less information regarding the pattern of response elicited when two or three functionally different groups are excited simultaneously. However, among the integrative neural mechanisms which are now known to play an important role

in the reflex control of the cardiovascular system are those brought about by changes in pulmonary ventilation. These will be discussed here and will be illustrated by considering two examples: first, the control of heart rate and systemic vascular resistance by the peripheral arterial chemoreceptors, the carotid and aortic bodies, under conditions in which pulmonary ventilation is increased; and, secondly, the mechanisms underlying the cardiac and systemic vascular components of the diving response, a pattern of response in which respiration temporarily ceases.

There are a number of ways by which respiration — both cyclic changes in breathing and sustained changes in alveolar ventilation — can exert effects on the cardiovascular system. Briefly, they are: (i) cyclic changes in respiration producing mechanical effects through variations in intrathoracic pressure; (ii) the cyclic changes in intrathoracic pressure resulting in alterations in transmural pressure in intrathoracic blood vessels and cardiac chambers, thereby altering the discharge frequency of vascular and cardiac receptors in the cardiopulmonary area (see Chapter 5); (iii) changes in blood gases having a direct action on peripheral blood vessels, thereby altering peripheral vascular resistance and the regional distribution of systemic blood flow; (iv) alterations in arterial blood gases affecting the discharge from peripheral arterial chemoreceptors, thereby initiating carotid and aortic body chemoreceptor reflexes that affect respiration, the heart and peripheral vascular resistance; and (v) both cyclic changes and sustained changes in respiration modifying the effectiveness of incoming signals to the central nervous system from

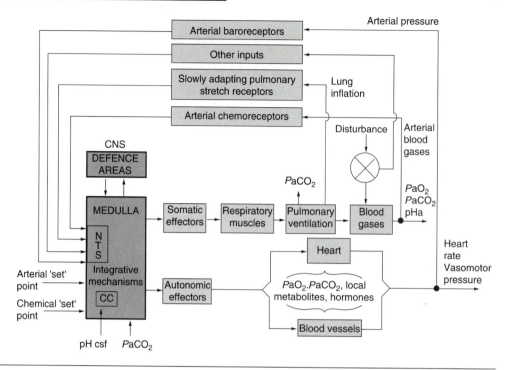

Fig. 1. **Some aspects of the control of the respiratory and cardiovascular systems by the arterial baroreceptors and chemoreceptors with some other inputs to the nervous system by which the integration between the two systems takes place**

Abbreviations used: csf, cerebrospinal fluid; CC, central chemoreceptors; CNS, central nervous system; NTS, nucleus tractus solitarius.

certain cardiovascular receptors, e.g. arterial baroreceptors, carotid body chemoreceptors and cardiac C-fibre endings. These respiratory effects are brought about through alterations in central inspiratory drive and changes in the input from slowly adapting pulmonary stretch receptors and will result in neural effects on heart rate and peripheral vascular resistance.

In this chapter, only the last of the above-mentioned mechanisms is to be considered, but a detailed discussion of the others is to be found elsewhere [1]. In that article the converse situation is also discussed, namely, the ways by which changes in the cardiovascular system can affect respiration.

As a first step, consideration will be given to the central respiratory and pulmonary reflex control of heart rate and systemic vascular resistance, the two neural mechanisms that are largely responsible for the effects of changes in respiration on the cardiovascular system.

Neurogenic effects of phasic changes in respiration on the cardiovascular system

Heart rate

The two basic mechanisms by which cyclic and maintained changes in respiration affect heart rate can be introduced by a brief historical account of respiratory sinus arrhythmia.

Carl Ludwig first described the respiratory variations in heart rate in 1847 [1]; during the phase of inspiration there is acceleration of the heart, followed by slowing during the expiratory phase. Respiratory sinus arrhythmia occurs in many mammalian species, including adult and newborn humans, marine mammals, and also in reptiles and fish. Following Ludwig's description, almost a century elapsed during which the mechanisms underlying respiratory sinus arrhythmia were surrounded in controversy. Early workers were agreed, however, that the arrhythmia was abolished by division of the cervical vagus nerves, which provided evidence as to its neural origin. Evidence for two main hypothesis evolved: first, a central mechanism whereby there was an 'overflow' or an 'irradiation' of impulses from the respiratory centres to the 'cardioinhibitory centre', thereby diminishing cardiac vagal tone. Secondly, a mechanism by which the tachycardia accompanying the inspiratory phase of the respiratory cycle was reflex in origin, resulting from stimulation of receptors in the lower airways by an increase in volume of the lungs. It was Anrep and his colleagues who later demonstrated convincingly that, in fact, both views were correct and that the central and pulmonary reflex mechanisms acted in concert during the respiratory cycle. To demonstrate these mechanisms they used the innervated heart–lung preparation in the dog, which consists essentially of a Starling heart–lung preparation with a facility for maintaining the blood flow to the brain of the animal. Inflation of the lungs in the absence of central inspiratory neuronal drive caused acceleration of the heart, which occurred independently of the sympathetic supply to the heart. The response was abolished, however, by selective denervation of the lungs, establishing the pulmonary origin of the reflex. Central inspiratory drive, as indicated by the phrenic nerve activity, also caused tachycardia and this response occurred while the lungs were maintained temporarily at their end-expiratory level, to exclude the pulmonary reflex, or after lung denervation.

Subsequent work has confirmed that both central and pulmonary reflex mechanisms are involved in respiratory sinus arrhythmia and that the efferent pathway is largely vagal in both animals and man [1,2]. It has also been established that an important factor in the demonstration of respiratory sinus arrhythmia is the presence of cardiac vagal tone, i.e. resting activity in the cardiac vagal efferent fibres. This is understandable if the vagus is the main efferent pathway, since cardioacceleration can only be brought about by a reduction in pre-existing vagal efferent fibre activity. This accounts for the variation in the size of respiratory sinus arrhythmia in different species: it is quite striking in humans and in chloralose-anaesthetized or conscious, non-excited resting dogs; it is weak or absent in conscious cats, rabbits and rats. However, even in species where sinus arrhythmia is normally present, it is suppressed by those anaesthetic agents with vagolytic properties.

Other theories as to the origin of respiratory sinus arrhythmia have, nonetheless, emerged: a reflex arising from receptors in the right atrium; a local mechanism resulting from stretch of the sinu-atrial node; and oscillations in $PaCO_2$ and arterial pH. These are reviewed elsewhere [1], and probably play a minor part. However, the role of the arterial baroreceptors is important. This is not so much because of the associated changes in arterial blood pressure, which in any case cannot explain respiratory sinus arrhythmia on the basis of a baroreceptor reflex associated with the small change in blood pressure, but because the arterial baroreceptor reflex input–output relationship is not constant during the respiratory cycle. This point is discussed below in more detail. Furthermore, there is also evidence that variations in heart rate may not be associated with every breath, but may appear temporarily, such as after muscular exercise, as large periodic changes in relation to breath cycle in a ratio of 1:1, 1:2 or 1:3 [1]. In other cases, slow oscillations of heart rate can occur in the absence of respiratory movements. The exact mechanisms in these cases have still to be worked out.

Vascular

Stephen Hales was the first to notice, in 1733, that oscillations in the level of the arterial blood pressure occurred in phase with respiration [1]. Three types of oscillation are now recognized: (i) fluctuations in phase with each heart beat; (ii) fluctuations in phase with each respiratory cycle resulting from (a) the mechanical effects of the 'respiratory pump' causing phasic changes in venous return and cardiac output, and (b) vasomotor changes synchronous with respiration which are largely of central origin — these variations in blood pressure are specifically referred to as Traube–Hering waves; and (iii) fluctuations in blood pressure due to rhythmic variations in vasomotor tone engendered by oscillations in activity of central presympathetic neurones. These rhythmic changes in blood pressure occur independently of respiration, are always much slower in rate and are referred to as Mayer waves [1].

The directional change in blood pressure with each phase of the respiratory cycle in humans is variable depending on the rate and depth of breathing, the type of breathing (abdominal or thoracic), posture and the presence of respiratory sinus arrhythmia. A deep voluntary inspiration in normal subjects and patients with spinal injuries at different levels causes a reduction in blood flow through the finger, independently of associated changes in blood pressure, indicating vasoconstriction [1]. Vasoconstriction also occurs in arterioles and venules in the forearm and hand. These vascular responses are not due to a fall in $PaCO_2$ but the exact nervous pathways through which they are mediated are still unknown. More than one mechanism may be involved and these could include a centrally mediated action of inspiratory neurones affecting the presympathetic neurones; a reflex involving the medullary or supramedullary regions of the brain; or a spinal reflex. The site of the receptors is also unknown but it has been suggested they could lie in the thorax, chest wall or diaphragm. In the intact organism it is difficult to dissociate vasomotor responses that originate centrally from those that are reflexly mediated. In animal experiments it has been shown that there is an increase in activity in sympathetic nerves coincident with the phrenic discharge (see section entitled Nature of pulmonary receptors), and this still occurs in paralysed animals during temporary interruption of artificial respiration. Phasic changes in vasomotor tone, however, are difficult to detect because the frequency of respiration is high in relation to the response time of smooth muscle.

Of the respiratory reflex components affecting vascular resistance, probably the most important is that resulting from inflation of the lungs [1,2]. The consensus of opinion is that when the lungs are inflated from their expiratory level with volumes of air up to 1.5 times the normal tidal volume, either statically from a syringe or phasically with a pump, vasodilatation occurs in a number of vascular territories, such as the intact limb, skin, muscle, kidney and splanchnic vascular bed. The responses are due to a reduction in activity of sympathetic noradrenergic fibres, and specific vasodilator fibres do not appear to be involved. They are dependent on the integrity of the innervation of the lungs and the afferent pathway lies in the vagus nerves [1,2].

Nature of pulmonary receptors

There is still some discussion about the type of receptor in the lungs responsible for the tachycardia and vasodilatation occurring on inflation of the lungs. Three types of receptor are now recognized [3,4]. (i) Slowly adapting pulmonary stretch receptors connected to myelinated fibres, which subserve the Hering–Breuer respiratory reflex. They respond to changes in lung volume and rate of change of volume. (ii) Irritant receptors which are rapidly adapting, connected to myelinated fibres, and are activated by chemical and mechanical irritants, and by mechanical changes in the lungs (pneumothorax, atelectasis, pulmonary congestion and microembolism). Reflexly they evoke hyperpnoea and bronchoconstriction. (iii) Pulmonary C-fibre endings [also called alveolar nociceptive receptors and J receptors (juxtapulmonary capillary receptors)] connected to non-myelinated fibres. Reflexly they cause apnoea, followed by rapid shallow breathing, bradycardia and peripheral vasodilatation. The tachycardia and vasodilatation resulting from inflation of the lungs are evoked by sustained lung inflations using relatively small changes in pressure and volume, and are well-maintained responses, providing that various secondary reflex effects are excluded. It is most likely that the receptors concerned are the slowly adapting pulmonary stretch receptors.

The initiation of the responses during the phasic inflation could also be evoked partly by irritant receptors which are rapidly adapting. Stimulation of pulmonary C-fibres is evoked by large inflations of the lungs (i.e. two to three times the eupnoeic tidal volume), and this causes bradycardia and vasodilatation. Thus, with large lung-volume inflations, pulmonary C-fibres could be involved in the vasodilator responses.

Respiratory modulation of cardiovascular reflexes

It is beyond the scope of this chapter to discuss in any detail the central control of respiration and the autonomic control of the circulation, but comprehensive, up-to-date reviews have appeared on the organization of the respiratory centres [5] and on the central mechanisms controlling the heart and peripheral circulation [6,7] (Chapter 1). Only a few points relevant to this discussion will, therefore, be covered here.

Receptors and afferent pathways

In this chapter we are concerned largely with those afferents controlling respiration and the circulation that arise from receptors in the skin of the face, upper and lower airways, from baroreceptors in arteries and the cardio-pulmonary area, and from peripheral arterial chemoreceptors. Afferents from arterial baro-receptors and chemoreceptors run in the glos-sopharyngeal and vagus nerves, which have their cell bodies in the petrosal and nodose ganglia, respectively. Other vagal afferents from the cardiopulmonary area, including slowly adapting pulmonary stretch receptors and those travelling in the superior laryngeal nerve from receptors in the larynx, have their cell bodies in the nodose ganglion. The cell bodies of the trigeminal afferents lie in the trigeminal (semilunar) ganglion. The major site for the first synapse of most, if not all, afferent fibres from receptors innervated by glossopharyngeal and vagus nerves is within the confines of the nucleus of the tractus solitarius (NTS) located in the dorsomedial medulla (Fig. 2). This is an elongated nucleus which runs rostral–caudally. The NTS also receives some trigeminal nerve afferents. The central terminals of the carotid sinus and aortic nerve afferents in the cat and rabbit are located in a relatively restricted area of the NTS in the dorsomedial medulla in the region 0.5–3.0 mm rostral to the obex, the so-called intermediate zone (see Chapter 1, Fig. 8). Another of these subnuclei, the ventrolateral subnucleus, contains one of the major group-ings of respiratory neurones. Projections from the NTS have been traced to a number of struc-tures, including the nucleus ambiguus, the dor-

sal motor nucleus of the vagus, the lateral retic-ular formation and hypothalamus [8].

Preganglionic cardiac vagal motoneurones

The activities in cardiac vagal efferent fibres recorded in the cervical vagus nerve, or in intrathoracic branches of the nerve, characteris-tically show two distinct firing patterns: cardiac and respiratory [1]. The cardiac rhythm is in phase with the heart beat, the frequency of dis-charge increasing with the rising phase of the arterial blood pressure. These changes in fre-quency are generated by inputs from the arter-ial baroreceptors.

The respiratory component shows a reduc-tion in cardiac vagal efferent activity during the inspiratory phase of the respiratory cycle and is associated with tachycardia. This respiratory modulation persists after division of the cervi-cal vagus nerves caudal to the level of recording, indicating it is partly central in origin. In addi-tion, there is a pulmonary reflex component — inflation of the lungs reducing the discharge rate provided that the vagus nerves are intact. This respiratory-related rhythm is superim-posed on the cardiac rhythm, so that firing in the cardiac vagal efferent fibres is normally seen predominantly in the expiratory phase of respi-ration.

The cell bodies of the cardiac vagal efferent fibres reside mainly in the ventrolateral compo-nent of the nucleus ambiguus, e.g. in the cat, but also, in some species at least, in the dorsal motor nucleus of the vagus (Fig. 3; see also Chapter 1, Fig. 6). Vagal cardiomotor neurones in the nucleus ambiguus have small myelinated axons. On the other hand, axons from car-diomotor neurones in the dorsal motor nucleus of the vagus are mostly non-myelinated [9]. In the anaesthetized cat, cardiac vagal motoneu-rones show little spontaneous activity and this is in keeping with the low level of cardiac vagal tone found in this animal. In those neurones that show spontaneous activity, however, and in those induced to fire by application of exci-tant amino acids, the discharge could be corre-lated with the central inspiratory drive; they invariably fired during the expiratory phase of the respiratory cycle and were silent during the inspiratory phase. Their activity was greatest during the early part of expiration [6]. The activity of cardiac vagal motoneurones mirrors that in cardiac vagal efferent fibres and is con-sistent with the changes in heart rate.

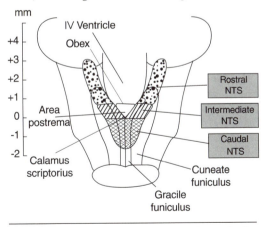

Fig. 2. **Diagrammatic representation of the dorsal medulla illustrating three zones of the NTS**

Reproduced with permission from Loewy [8].

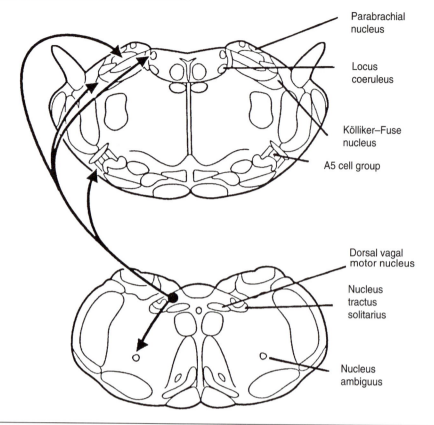

Parabrachial nucleus

Locus coeruleus

Kölliker–Fuse nucleus

A5 cell group

Dorsal vagal motor nucleus

Nucleus tractus solitarius

Nucleus ambiguus

Fig. 3. Diagram showing projections from the NTS to other nuclei in the lower brainstem
Reproduced with permission from Loewy [8].

Respiratory modulation of excitatory inputs to cardiac vagal motoneurones

In their studies on the baroreceptor reflex control of heart rate, Koepchen and colleagues demonstrated that an electrical stimulus to the carotid sinus nerve caused slowing of the heart, but only if the stimulus was timed to coincide with the expiratory phase of the respiratory cycle; a similar stimulus given in inspiration produced a much attenuated response [6]. This respiratory modulation of the effectiveness of the baroreceptor control of heart rate has been confirmed in cats, dogs and human subjects. Indeed, other excitatory inputs to cardiac vagal motoneurones from the carotid body chemo-receptors, receptors in the nasopharynx, trigeminal receptors in the skin of the face, receptors in the larynx and cardiac ventricular C-fibre endings are affected in a similar way [1,2]. There are three mechanisms by which this respiratory 'gating' of the excitatory inputs to

cardiac vagal motoneurones could take place: it could result from a gating of the inputs to the cardiac vagal motoneurones during inspiration, from respiratory-related changes in the excitability of the cardiac vagal motoneurones, or from a combination of the two. It was evident [6] that this apparent gating could not be explained by a presynaptic control of the central terminals of the baroreceptor afferents within the NTS, since the excitability of carotid sinus and aortic nerve afferent terminals did not alter in phase with central respiratory activity.

Studies of the events occurring in the cardiac vagal motoneurones situated in the nucleus ambiguus during the respiratory cycle indicated that neurones with a respiratory-related rhythm were involved. The firing pattern of the cardiac vagal motoneurones was the result of an inhibitory effect on their activity through an inspiratory-related inhibitory input, which was mediated by a muscarinic cholinergic synapse.

This inhibitory control of the cardiac vagal motoneurones involved a direct cholinergic mechanism from neurones with an inspiratory-related firing pattern (Fig. 4) [6]. Thus a central synaptic mechanism is responsible for the apparent gating of the baroreceptor input and on this basis provides an explanation for the phenomenon of respiratory sinus arrhythmia.

Lung stretch afferents terminate in the NTS where there is no evidence for any pre-synaptic interaction with baroreceptor afferents (see above). However, lung inflation fails to produce any obvious changes in the membrane potential in cardiomotor neurones, suggesting that lung-stretch modulation is mediated at a site(s) along the polysynaptic pathway between the NTS and the nucleus ambiguus (Fig. 4) [6].

These results on the respiratory modulation of excitatory inputs to cardiac vagal motoneurones are important in relation to the reflex control of heart rate. They mean that the effectiveness of several excitatory inputs from the carotid chemoreceptors, arterial barorecep-tors and cardiac C-fibres is dependent on the respiratory-related excitability of the cardiac vagal motoneurones (Fig. 4). This is illustrated in Fig. 5, which shows diagrammatically the effects of brief selective stimuli delivered to the carotid body chemoreceptors at different phases of the respiratory cycle. During the expiratory phase of respiration, they evoke slowing of the heart and an increase in cardiac vagal efferent fibre activity. When delivered during the inspiratory phase, they have little or no effect, or may sometimes cause tachycardia owing to the over-riding effect of the combina-tion of the central inspiratory neuronal activity and activity of lung stretch afferents [1,2].

Thus, in a situation where there is a concomitant increased inspiratory drive, the excitability of the cardiac vagal motoneurones will be reduced — with the consequence that

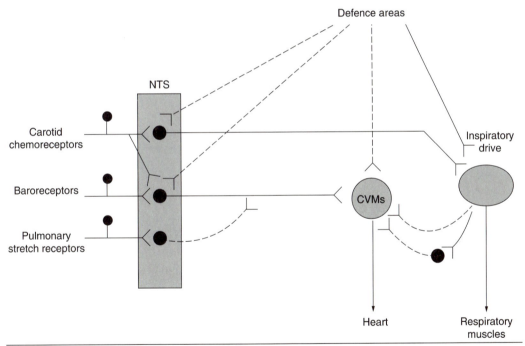

Fig. 4. **Diagram illustrating the control of the cardiac vagal motoneurones (CVMs) by barorecep-tor and chemoreceptor inputs, inspiratory drive, pulmonary stretch afferents and hypothalamic defence area**

The respiratory modulation of CVMs is brought about by two mechanisms. (i) Activity of central inspiratory neu-rones exerts an inhibitory control of the CVMs, either directly or through an inter-neurone. This inhibitory action is mediated by a cholinergic mechanism. (ii) Activity of slowly adapting pulmonary stretch receptors driven by inflation of the lungs exerts an inhibitory control of CVMs, probably through an action on the polysynaptic pathway between the NTS and CVMs. The inhibitory control of the CVMs and NTS by the hypothalamic defence area is mediated by GABA. Continuous lines, excitatory path-ways; dashed lines, inhibitory pathways.

the primary cardiac response, bradycardia, resulting from an excitatory input will be wholly or partly suppressed. Where the respiratory drive is reduced, the excitability of the cardiac vagal motoneurones will be increased, resulting in an enhancement of the effectiveness of the excitatory input to cardiac vagal motoneurones and of cardiac inhibition. These conditions are pertinent in the examples considered below concerning the respiratory integration of cardiovascular reflexes during stimulation of the peripheral arterial chemoreceptors and in the diving response.

Phasic respiratory modulation of excitatory inputs to respiratory neurones

Also important in the integrative control of the cardiovascular system by changes in respiration is the phasic modulation of excitatory inputs to

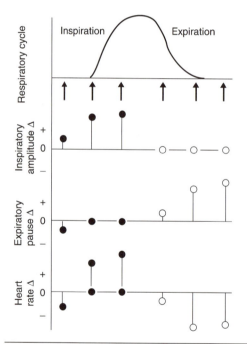

Brief stimulation of carotid body

Fig. 5. Modulation by phasic changes in respiration of the respiratory and heart rate responses to brief stimuli applied to the carotid body chemoreceptors by agents injected into a common carotid artery

Stimuli were delivered to the carotid body during the inspiratory (●) and expiratory (○) phase of the respiratory cycle, as indicated by the arrows. Data taken from [16,18] and M. de B. Daly, unpublished work.

respiratory neurones. The reflex respiratory response to brief stimuli applied to the carotid body chemoreceptors depends on the phase of the respiratory cycle in which the stimuli are delivered (Fig. 5) [1]. When excitatory stimuli are delivered during the inspiratory phase of the cycle, an increase in the size of the ongoing inspiratory activity occurs. When the stimuli are delivered during the expiratory phase, however, there is either no effect on respiration or a prolongation of expiration and sometimes an active expiratory effort.

Influence of the hypothalamus

The NTS also receives an input from the hypothalamic defence area (see Chapter 3). Stimulation of areas of the hypothalamus that elicit the alerting or defence response causes suppression of the baroreceptor–cardiac reflex. One mechanism by which this occurs is the inhibition of NTS neurones that are normally excited during baroreceptor activation. This inhibition involves a chloride-dependent inhibitory postsynaptic potential and is mediated by a GABAergic synapse (GABA, γ-aminobutyric acid). There is also evidence that stimulation of the defence area can exert a direct inhibitory action on cardiac vagal motoneurones in the nucleus ambiguus. This dual effect of controlling the efficacy of the reflex inputs (at the level of the NTS) and of the excitability of the preganglionic vagal and sympathetic neurones may provide a means of modifying both the gain and the set point of cardiovascular reflexes (Fig. 4) [10].

Sympathetic outflow

The preganglionic neurones in the intermediolateral cell column of the spinal cord are controlled by a number of spinal and bulbo-spinal excitatory and inhibitory pathways [8,11,12] (see also Chapter 1). There is normally ongoing activity in sympathetic vasomotor fibres, giving rise to vasomotor tone in peripheral vessels. The possible regions in the brainstem and higher parts of the central nervous system responsible for generating this tone are discussed elsewhere [12] (see also Chapter 1). Records of activity in various pre- and postganglionic sympathetic fibres reveal several periodicities. (i) Waves of 2–6 Hz synchronized to the arterial pressure wave. The discharge is probably generated centrally and then entrained to the cardiac cycle by the pulse-synchronous baroreceptor afferent activity. (ii) An oscillation in phase with the central inspiratory drive, as indicated by the phrenic nerve discharge. The exact relationship is complex and may be species dependent but, nevertheless, a clear relation to one or other of the phases of the respiratory cycle is usually seen. In the cat, for example, increasing sympathetic activity in many neurones occurs with a peak frequency in inspiration and with a minimum frequency during expiration. A few neurones show a peak frequency during expiration, while in others there is no respiratory modulation. Again, the respiratory component of the sympathetic discharge can be influenced reflexly by inflation of the lungs. Lung inflation inhibits sympathetic activity in two ways: first, by inhibiting central inspiratory drive through the Hering–Breuer reflex, thereby inhibiting the inspiratory-related activity from the inspiratory to sym-pathetic neurones, and, secondly, through pathways different from those that affect the respiratory centres. This means that during

the inspiratory phase of the respiratory cycle there are two different and opposing mechanisms affecting sympathetic activity. On the one hand, there is a centrally-induced inspiratory activity increasing the discharge and, simultaneously on the other, an augmented discharge in pulmonary stretch afferents driven by inflation of the lungs, which inhibits sympathetic activity. The magnitude of the respiratory modulation of the sympathetic discharge will, therefore, be determined by the relative strengths of the central and pulmonary reflex mechanisms. It will also be governed by the prevailing physiological conditions; thus, during positive pressure artificial respiration, the central and lung inflation reflex components may be out of phase, leading to an altered respiratory pattern of activity in sympathetic efferent fibres.

There is still much to be learned about the central pathways by which respiratory modulation of sympathetic activity is brought about. A group of neurones in the rostral ventrolateral medulla (see Chapter 1, Figs. 2, 4 and 5) may be involved. These may, at least in part, be responsible for generating vasomotor tone. The pattern of discharge of these neurones is in many respects similar to that in sympathetic fibres. They show similar respiratory-related firing patterns and are affected in a similar way by

inputs from arterial baroreceptors, peripheral arterial chemoreceptors and excitation of superior laryngeal afferents.

Respiratory modulation of inputs to the presympathetic neurones

The effects of excitatory inputs from cardiovascular receptors on sympathetic nerve activity and sympathetic nerve responses are dependent on the phase of respiration in which they are delivered, as in the case of the vagus nerve responses (Fig. 5). Thus the effects of arterial baroreceptor and chemoreceptor stimulation, on sympathetic nerve activity and on the sympathetic control of heart rate and vascular resistance, are greater during expiration than inspiration. These effects are due largely to the inhibitory effect of lung stretch afferents during the inspiratory phase of the respiratory cycle but also to a central phenomenon. Hyperventilation at constant $PaCO_2$ reduces sympathetic activity, partly because of a reflex from the lungs. During suppression of respiration (apnoea) produced by excitation of the central cut end of a superior laryngeal nerve, the vasoconstrictor response to excitation of the carotid bodies is enhanced.

The evidence indicates, therefore, that, as with reflex vagal responses, reflex sympathetic effects to excitation of cardiovascular afferents undergo respiratory modulation, being wholly or partly suppressed during the inspiratory phase of the respiratory cycle, owing to a central and pulmonary reflex mechanism. As will become evident in the next two sections, these same mechanisms play an important role in the integrative control of the cardiovascular system during stimulation of the peripheral arterial chemoreceptors and in the diving response.

▶ Preganglionic cardiac vagal motoneurones in the nucleus ambiguus exhibit cardiac and respiratory rhythms which are mirrored in cardiac vagal efferent fibres.
▶ The activity of cardiac vagal motoneurones is rhythmically inhibited by two 'respiratory' mechanisms: activity of central inspiratory neurones and activity of slowly adapting pulmonary stretch receptors during the inspiratory phase of the respiratory cycle.

▶ During the inspiratory phase of respiration the cardiac vagal motoneurones are refractory to incoming excitatory impulses from arterial baroreceptors, arterial chemoreceptors and cardiac ventricular C-fibres. Thus it is only during expiration that the full expression of these excitatory inputs causing bradycardia is seen. The phasic modulation of excitability of the cardiac vagal motoneurones accounts for respiratory sinus arrhythmia.

▶ There is also a respiratory modulation of inputs to the central sympathetic neurones.

Integrative control of the respiratory and cardiovascular systems by the peripheral arterial chemoreceptors

The peripheral arterial chemoreceptors are represented by the carotid and aortic bodies. Whereas the carotid bodies have been found in all mammals in which they have been sought, the aortic bodies are not present in all mammalian species. It was perhaps fortuitous that the dog was used in studies in which J.-F. Heymans and C. Heymans (father and son) discovered the functions of the aortic bodies in 1927 [13]. These chemoreceptors are abundant in this species and in the cat too. Their distribution in the thorax is diffuse, in contrast to the carotid bodies, and they are therefore sometimes referred to as thoracic chemoreceptors. On the other hand, in the rabbit, rat and mouse, the aortic bodies are absent or at least very sparsely distributed; there is very little information in this respect so far as the non-human primate and man are concerned. The species differences in the mass of aortic chemoreceptor tissue are important when quantitative studies are made of the reflex responses evoked from the carotid and aortic bodies. Furthermore, the differences of the distribution in those species possessing aortic bodies means that their blood supply is derived from several parent vessels and, as a consequence, it is difficult to stimulate them selectively by chemical agents without at the same time affecting other sensory nerve endings.

Where quantitative studies of the reflex control of respiration by the peripheral arterial chemoreceptors have been made in species known to possess aortic bodies (e.g. the dog),

the carotid bodies play the greater role in the reflex control of breathing by a factor of about seven [2]. The situation is probably the same in man because in patients whose carotid bodies were surgically removed for therapeutic reasons, the ventilatory response to hypoxia was drastically reduced or abolished.

Cardiovascular responses to stimulation of the peripheral arterial chemoreceptors: role of changes in respiration

A comprehensive survey of the literature on this subject is to be found in the reviews elsewhere [1,2].

Carotid bodies

In spontaneously breathing anaesthetized animals, stimulation of the isolated perfused carotid bodies with hypoxic blood causes an increase in pulmonary ventilation but variable changes in heart rate, arterial blood pressure, cardiac output and total peripheral and regional vascular resistances. For example, in the dog, tachycardia or bradycardia occurred together with vasodilatation or vasoconstriction. In the monkey, there was a predominance of tachycardia and vasodilatation, in the cat the responses were largely bradycardia and vasoconstriction and in the rat, tachycardia and vasoconstriction. These variable responses were unlikely to be due to differences in species because they could occur at different times in the same animal. It seemed more probable that they were complicated by other reflex or humoral effects which occurred secondarily to the stimulus to the carotid chemoreceptors (Fig. 1).

A number of observations indicated that an important secondary factor was the increase in pulmonary ventilation occurring contemporaneously. The following evidence indicates that, when respiration is prevented from changing, bradycardia and peripheral vasoconstriction occur and these responses probably represent the direct or primary cardiac and vascular responses from the carotid bodies; the tachycardia and peripheral vasodilatation are secondary to the hyperventilation.

— When stimulation of the carotid bodies caused an acceleration of the heart, the same stimulus carried out with controlled pulmonary ventilation invariably resulted in bradycardia. Controlled ventilation unmasked a bradycardia when, under conditions of spontaneous respiration, no change in rate occurred. Controlled pulmonary ventilation was equally effective in modifying the vascular responses to excitation of the carotid bodies, vasodilator responses in spontaneously breathing animals being converted to vasoconstriction during controlled ventilation.

— In the conscious dog, brief stimulations of the carotid body resulted in an increase in pulmonary ventilation, an initial bradycardia followed by tachycardia, and an initial peripheral vasoconstriction followed by vasodilatation. When the test was repeated during controlled pulmonary ventilation, both the cardioinhibitory and vasoconstrictor responses were enhanced, while the tachycardia and vasodilatation were abolished. In this instance, the 'respiratory' secondary effects modulating the cardiovascular system were not prepotent in the spontaneously breathing animal.

— All these results were obtained under conditions in which arterial baroreceptor reflexes resulting from changes in blood pressure could be excluded.

— Using a different experimental approach to this problem, the role of the carotid bodies was evaluated in the control of heart rate during systemic hypoxia [1,2]. In many species, although not in all, tachycardia occurred when hypoxia was induced by inhalation of a gas mixture containing a lowered concentration of oxygen. If, during the period of systemic hypoxia, the carotid chemoreceptor 'drive' was withdrawn by selectively perfusing the chemoreceptors with oxygenated blood (the animal remaining hypoxic), no change in heart rate or a further cardiac acceleration occurred independently of the change in breathing. This indicates the tachycardia of hypoxia could not have been due to the effect of carotid body stimulation; indeed, the chemoreceptor contribution under these conditions is sometimes to suppress, at least in part, the cardioaccelerator response.

Further evidence supporting the fact that the tachycardia of systemic hypoxia is not due primarily to stimulation of the carotid bodies has been obtained in man. Mild hypoxia causes acceleration of the heart. If the subject is then given 100% O_2 to breathe, to rapidly increase his PaO_2 and thereby withdraw the carotid body drive, a further acceleration of the heart

takes place with the peak response coinciding with the estimated pulmonary capillary–carotid body circulation time. Thus, in both laboratory animals and man, stimulation of the carotid bodies in the absence of changes in breathing causes bradycardia. This response is mediated largely by way of the vagus nerves.

There are at least three mechanisms by which an increase in pulmonary ventilation suppresses or even reverses the bradycardia and vasoconstriction resulting from stimulation of the carotid bodies: (i) an increase in central respiratory drive; (ii) increased activity of slowly adapting pulmonary stretch receptors; and (iii) a reduction in $PaCO_2$ acting, at least in part, centrally. It is usually sufficient to control the two neurogenic components to unmask the primary cardiac and vascular responses (Fig. 6). Therefore, these results fall into line with those concerning the mechanisms underlying respiratory sinus arrhythmia.

The pattern of response to selective stimulation of the carotid bodies does, however, depend on the anaesthetic used. Chloralose, urethane and barbiturates prevent activation of the brainstem defence areas from afferent inputs, including that from the carotid bodies, which is in contrast to the steroid anaesthetic alphaxalone–alphadalone (Althesin, Saffan). This latter agent produces adequate anaesthesia and yet allows the autonomic components of the alerting stage of the defence response to predominate (see Chapter 3). These include tachycardia, renal and mesenteric vasoconstriction, and vasodilatation in skeletal muscle. These effects are not secondary to the accompanying hyperventilation. When the alerting response is evoked by stimulation of the carotid bodies, these responses are superimposed upon the primary and secondary effects that are seen under chloralose, urethane or barbiturate anaesthesia. As the depth of Saffan anaesthesia is increased, carotid body stimulation evokes a pattern of response comparable with that seen under the three other anaesthetic agents.

In the conscious animal, stimulation of the carotid bodies can cause hyperventilation, bradycardia and peripheral vasoconstriction, as described above, the cardiac and vascular responses being potentiated when respiration is controlled or inhibited reflexly [1,2]. These responses are, therefore, more like those obtained under chloralose, urethane and barbiturates than under light Saffan anaesthesia.

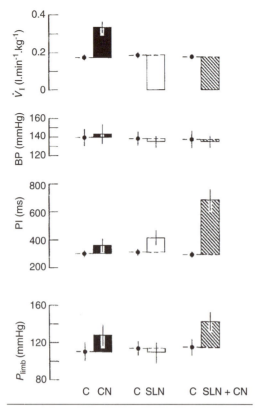

Fig. 6. Comparison of the cardiac and vascular responses to stimulation of the carotid body chemoreceptors during normal breathing and during a reflexly induced apnoea evoked by electrical stimulation of the central cut end of a superior laryngeal nerve

Paired data (peak values, mean ± S.E.M.) from six series tests in five cats anaesthetized with a mixture of chloralose and urethane. A hindlimb was vascularly isolated and perfused with blood at constant flow. The three panels include the effects of stimulation of the carotid chemoreceptors with intracarotid injections of sodium cyanide alone (CN), electrical stimulation of a superior laryngeal nerve alone (SLN), and in combination (SLN+CN). C, control values. Where no standard error bar is shown, it is smaller than the size of the symbol. Abbreviations used: V_I, respiratory minute volume; BP, mean arterial blood pressure; PI, pulse interval; P_{limb}, hindlimb perfusion pressure. Reproduced with permission from [26].

However, under some circumstances tachycardia and peripheral vasodilatation with behavioural alerting can be evoked (see Chapter 3). The explanation may be that the threshold for evoking the bradycardia and peripheral vaso-constriction through bulbo-pontine neurones is lower than that for evoking the components of the alerting response. Alternatively, under Saffan anaesthesia, transmission in inhibitory inputs to the defence areas is impaired or removed, thereby enabling the full expression of the autonomic responses of the defence areas.

Aortic bodies

This group of chemoreceptors is less accessible to experimentation, but it is evident that their stimulation by hypoxic hypercapnic blood causes only a small increase in respiration relative to that evoked by stimulation of the carotid bodies with blood of the same gaseous composition [2]. When respiration is controlled artificially, the cardiovascular responses include a weak bradycardia or tachycardia and invariably a striking increase in total systemic vascular resistance and in vascular resistance in the abdominal viscera. Quantitatively, the size of the systemic vasoconstrictor response is approximately the same as that evoked by excitation of the carotid bodies with hypoxic blood of the same gaseous composition [2]. These reflex vascular responses, like those elicited by stimulation of the carotid bodies, are subject to respiratory modulation, at least by excitation of pulmonary stretch afferents. Quantitative information, however, is still lacking.

▶ Stimulation of the carotid body chemoreceptors causes reflex bradycardia and vasoconstriction in most vascular beds. These responses, however, are often suppressed or even reversed by the concomitant hyperventilation.

▶ The mechanisms by which the increased ventilation opposes these chemoreceptor cardiovascular responses include an increased central inspiratory neuronal activity and increased activity of lung stretch afferents.

▶ These respiratory–cardiovascular integrative mechanisms also operate in conditions, such as systemic hypoxia, which account (at least in part) for the variable cardiovascular responses seen in this condition.

▶ The full expression of the carotid chemoreceptor primary cardiac and vascular responses is seen in conditions in which respiration is inhibited either centrally or reflexly by another input. These responses are also seen in the conscious animal. The primary cardiac and vascular responses elicited by stimulation of the carotid bodies are also opposed by excitation of defence areas that give rise to the alerting response under Saffan anaesthesia.

The diving response

This term is applied to a pattern of response that consists essentially of three effects: apnoea, bradycardia and selective peripheral vasoconstriction. Other cardiovascular effects include a reduction in cardiac output and variable changes in blood pressure. Vasoconstriction occurs in virtually all regions of the body, with the exception of the cerebral circulation, and is mediated by sympathetic noradrenergic fibres. This means that the reduced cardiac output is redistributed towards the brain.

The term 'diving reflex' has sometimes been used to describe this pattern of response, which implies that the respiratory and cardiovascular changes are the result of a single reflex. As will become evident, this is not so; the response pattern is due to a number of reflexes, with the cessation of breathing playing a dominant role in the integration of the cardiovascular effects. The term diving response would, therefore, seem to be a more appropriate one to use. As the term implies, this pattern of response is seen in breath-hold diving and in these circumstances is triggered by the immersion of the face in water through stimulation of receptors in the skin of the face innervated by the trigeminal nerves. Immersion of other parts of the body does not elicit these responses, but instead leads to hyperventilation, tachycardia and a rise in blood pressure. The diving response can also be elicited in other ways, such as by stimulation of receptors in the upper airways (nasal mucosa and larynx) which are not involved in the responses to breath-hold diving. In fact, the first description of the diving response was given in 1870 by Kratschmer (see [14]), who studied the effects of excitation of

the nasal mucosa by tobacco smoke in the conscious rabbit. The responses can be very dramatic (Fig. 7). A number of irritant gases and vapours passed through the nose have the same effect. The respiratory and cardiovascular responses are reflex in nature because they are abolished by applying a local anaesthetic to the nasal mucosa or by division of the trigeminal nerves. Receptors in the larynx can be stimulated by a number of chemical agents and by mechanical stimuli. There is now extensive literature on the diving response, which has been comprehensively reviewed in a number of publications relating to breath-hold diving [1,14,15], reflexes from the nasal mucosa [1,14] and reflexes from the larynx [17]. It occurs in terrestrial mammals, including adult and newborn humans, marine mammals, reptiles, amphibia and some avian species.

The diving response, from whatever cause, serves a number of functions. First, it provides a defence mechanism against asphyxia in that it helps to conserve oxygen and to ensure that the brain preferentially receives a supply of blood when the organism as a whole is deprived of oxygen. Not all organs of the body are equally tolerant of a temporary deficiency of oxygen; the brain is far less able to tolerate low oxygen tensions than other tissues, such as skin, skeletal muscle and viscera, which can survive by anaerobic glycolysis. The redistribution of the reduced cardiac output by vasoconstriction in these regions ensures that the brain receives preferentially the limited stores of oxygen in the blood. Secondly, apnoea, which is at least partly reflexly engendered, acts as a defence mechanism for the lungs in that noxious gases and vapours are prevented access to the lower airways. Thirdly, the diving response is functionally useful in that, in those marine animals in which it is particularly well-developed, it allows a longer period of time for foraging for food in water than would otherwise be possible. Although in these animals the oxygen stores in the blood are relatively larger than in terrestrial mammals, on account of their increased haemoglobin concentration, oxygen capacity and blood volume, they are inadequate to sustain them during prolonged dives at the pre-dive rate of oxygen consumption.

Breath-hold diving
The main features of the respiratory and cardiovascular responses to face immersion in man

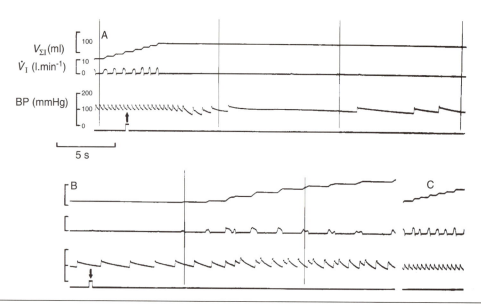

Fig. 7. The effects of stimulation of upper airways receptors (nasopharyngeal) by cigarette smoke in the conscious rabbit between arrows ↑↓

(A) and (B) are continuous records. Between (B) and (C) is an interval of 1 min. Records from (top): $V_{\Sigma I}$, accumulated inspiratory volume; $\dot{V}_I$, inspiratory flow; BP, arterial blood pressure. Time marker, 10 s; time calibration, 5 s. Note: (i) prolonged apnoea; (ii) cardiac asystole lasting 10.7 s; and (iii) the gradual reduction in the slope of the 'run off' of the arterial pressure wave, indicating increasing peripheral vasoconstriction. Towards the end of the period of cardiac asystole, the pressure wave remains almost horizontal at a pressure of 100 mmHg. Reproduced with permission from [27].

include apnoea, bradycardia, a small rise in systolic and diastolic blood pressure and a reduction in forearm blood flow. The calculated forearm vascular resistance (mean arterial blood pressure/blood flow) is therefore increased. By comparison, however, the responses are much more striking in marine mammals: heart rate and cardiac output fall by as much as 80% and the peripheral vasoconstriction is intense, the blood flow in the abdominal aorta virtually ceasing. This means that in a prolonged dive these animals become a 'heart–lung–head' preparation. The maximum duration of dives in these animals varies from 25 min in the harbour seal *Phoca vitulina richardsi* to 120 min in the Southern elephant seal *Mirounga leonina*, although most dives are of much shorter duration. This compares with maximum breath-hold times in man of 0.75–1.5 min, that is without prior hyperventilation or oxygen breathing. Breath-hold dives are associated with a progressive fall in PaO_2 and a rise in $PaCO_2$, the changes being more evident the longer the dive. In prolonged dives in marine mammals, values for PaO_2 less than 20 mmHg (2.67 kPa) and for $PaCO_2$ up to 100 mmHg (13.3 kPa) have been recorded, a degree of hypoxaemia and hypercapnia which causes vigorous carotid body chemoreceptor activity [19].

Integrative mechanisms concerning the respiratory and cardiovascular responses

The bradycardia and selective vasoconstriction occurring during breath-hold diving are the result of complex nervous and humoral effects, the full expression of the reflex responses being entirely dependent on the concomitant change in respiration, i.e. apnoea, but they are undoubtedly subject to modification by higher parts of the nervous system. A central feature of the physiology of breath-hold diving, as will be evident from the discussion that follows, is the cessation of external respiration during the period of submersion, with the progressive development of asphyxia (a combination of arterial hypoxaemia and hypercapnia). It will also become apparent that the apnoea plays an important role in the integration of the cardiovascular responses that occur as part of the diving response. It is appropriate, therefore, to discuss next the various inputs to the nervous system that are involved in the diving response.

Trigeminal receptors

The receptors that trigger the diving response are those situated in the skin of the face innervated by the ophthalmic and maxillary branches of the trigeminal nerves. Reflexes from the nasal mucosa are not normally involved in the responses to face immersion in water. In marine mammals, for example, water is prevented from gaining access to the nasal passages by contraction of the muscles surrounding the external nares. In man, the combination of face immersion and breath-holding causes a greater bradycardia than either face immersion or breath-holding alone. Furthermore, when the face is removed from the water while the subject continues to hold his breath, the heart rate and forearm blood flow return towards the control levels existing before the test commenced. Thus it is only the combination of apnoea and face immersion that causes the maximum cardiac and vascular responses.

Arterial baroreceptors

During breath-hold diving, the arterial blood pressure either does not change or rises slightly. Because there is an accompanying marked reduction in heart rate, it means that the baroreflex control of pulse interval is reset towards bradycardia at a given level of blood pressure (Fig. 8) [20]. Fig. 8 also shows that the dive causes an increase in the gain or sensitivity of the baroreflex control of pulse interval (change in pulse interval per mmHg change in systolic blood pressure). Similar changes in the setting and gain of the reflex were found to occur on excitation of the receptors in the nasal mucosa.

There are three possible explanations for these changes. First, cessation of respiratory activity leads to a fuller expression of the input from arterial baroreceptors to cardiac vagal motoneurones. This change in the baroreceptor input–output relationship could, in fact, explain the finding in man that, during face immersion, there is no correlation between the changes in heart rate and arterial blood pressure. Secondly, an increase in activity of the carotid bodies by

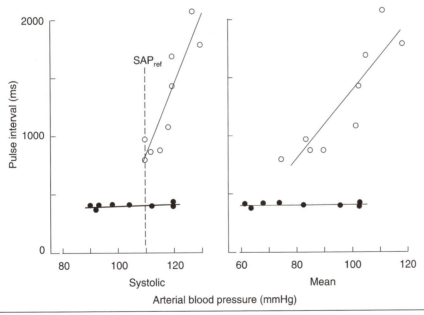

Fig. 8. Plots of pulse interval against systolic and mean arterial blood pressure immediately before and during the rise in pressure induced by the injection of phenylephrine (10 μg·kg⁻¹ i.v.) before and during a dive in an anaesthetized seal

●, control non-dive state; ○, during experimental dive (face immersion). Slopes of regression lines for pulse interval on systolic pressure are 0.16 ms ·mmHg⁻¹ (r = 0.12; P>0.6) and 29.6 ms ·mmHg⁻¹ (r = 0.9; P<0.05), respectively. Abbreviation used: SAP$_{ref}$, reference systolic blood pressure. Reproduced with permission from [20].

arterial hypoxaemia and hypercapnia elicits a primary reflex bradycardia. Thirdly, a combination of the two could cause the changes.

Carotid body chemoreceptors

It had been suggested that the bradycardia occurring on head immersion in some diving animals might be due to stimulation of the peripheral arterial chemoreceptors by hypoxaemia and hypercapnia occurring as a result of the apnoea. If this were true, however, an explanation had to be sought as to why the peripheral chemoreceptor drive did not (at the same time) provide a stimulus to breathe and compel the animal to emerge from the water. Evidence in favour of a chemoreceptor contribution to the cardiovascular component of the diving response was provided by a number of different studies. Electroneurograms of chemoreceptor fibres in the carotid sinus nerve show that nerve fibre activity gradually increases. Such chemoreceptor activity normally reflexly increases pulmonary ventilation and has variable effects on heart rate and peripheral vascular resistance. However, when it is associated with apnoea — induced reflexly by excitation of the receptors in the skin of the face — conditions are optimal for elicitation of the primary cardiac (bradycardia) and vascular (vasoconstrictor) responses to stimulation of the carotid bodies due to suppression of the secondary respiratory effects [1,2,4].

Fig. 6 demonstrates the contrasting effects of increased carotid body activity on respiration and pulse interval during normal breathing and during a reflexly induced apnoea. During normal breathing, stimulation of the carotid bodies causes an increase in pulmonary ventilation and slowing of the heart. When, however, the same stimulus is applied during a reflexly induced apnoea, there is no effect on respiration, but an enhanced cardioinhibitory response occurs. The counterpart of this experiment is shown in Fig. 5. Here, brief carotid body stimuli delivered during the expiratory phase of respiration only had the effect of prolonging expiration and causing bradycardia. During the asphyxial stage of a breath-hold dive, therefore, the magnitude of the inhibitory effect on respiration is such that it not only suppresses the excitatory effect of stimulation of the carotid bodies, but that of the increased level of $PaCO_2$ acting centrally as well. A stage must eventually be reached when the sum total

of the excitatory effects on the inspiratory neurones predominates to provide a compelling urge to breathe, although the exact mechanisms are not known. The relationships of the various inputs to cardiac vagal motoneurones during the diving response are shown diagrammatically in Fig. 9.

The evidence concerning the role of the carotid bodies in the responses to face immersion is shown in Fig. 10 [19]. Face immersion caused apnoea and bradycardia, with little change in arterial blood pressure. When the carotid body drive was withdrawn 105 s after face immersion, heart rate was restored to its control level. Bradycardia occurred on re-introducing to the carotid bodies hypoxic hypercapnic blood from the animal's carotid artery to restore the chemoreceptor drive, but there was no effect on breathing; the apnoea persisted. Finally, on emersion, there was resumption of breathing and acceleration of the heart to its pre-dive level. The control experiment, of substituting arterialized blood for the animal's own blood in the carotid body perfusate immediately after commencing the dive and before any hypoxaemia occurred, had no effect on heart rate. This experiment demonstrates a number of points: first, that excitation of the carotid bodies contributes to the bradycardia and also to the hindlimb vasoconstriction [M. de B. Daly, R. Elsner and J.E. Angell-James (1975), unpublished work] but only during the asphyxial stage of the dive. Secondly, during face immersion, apnoea persists even in the presence of asphyxia, and hence an increased drive to respiration occurs not only from the resulting carotid chemoreceptor activity but also from the elevated level of $PaCO_2$ acting on central respiratory neurones. The contrasting effects of the carotid chemoreceptor drive to respiration and heart rate are shown in Fig. 10 (columns 3 and 4). The apnoea in the expiratory position is maintained by the powerful trigeminal nerve inhibitory input to the respiratory centres, which in turn allows the full expression of the cardiac response resulting from the excitatory input to the cardiac vagal motoneurones. Finally, during the dive, the trigeminal input appears to undergo differentiation in that at the onset of face immersion it is responsible for the initiation of both the apnoea and bradycardia. During the asphyxial stage of the dive, however, the apnoea is maintained by the trigeminal input, whereas the bradycardia is maintained

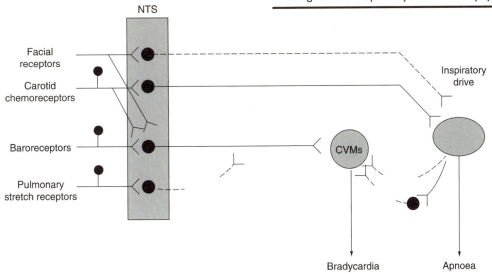

Fig. 9. Diagrammatic representation of the control of the cardiac vagal motoneurones (CVMs) during the diving response elicited by the excitation of receptors in the skin of the face by immersion in water

The inhibitory input to inspiratory drive causes apnoea. The full expression of excitatory inputs to the CVMs from the facial receptors (innervated by the trigeminal nerves), carotid bodies (stimulated during the progressive asphyxial stage of the diving response) and arterial baroreceptors is now possible in the absence of inhibitory inputs from the inspiratory neurones and lung stretch afferents. The latter is indicated in the diagram by interruption of the relevant pathways. The inhibitory effects of the trigeminal input to inspiratory neurones predominates over the excitatory effect of stimulation of the chemo-receptors and the central effects of the rising $PaCO_2$. Eventually, however, a respiratory breakthrough occurs. Continuous lines, excitatory pathways; dashed lines, inhibitory pathways.

solely by the carotid bodies. The exact mechanisms involved here are not at present clear.

On emersion from the water, there is an immediate removal of the trigeminal inhibitory input to the respiratory centres, leading to the resumption of breathing. With the first breath there is acceleration of the heart, which is probably determined largely by the increased refractoriness of the cardiac vagal motoneurones to excitatory effects from the trigeminal receptors, the carotid chemoreceptors and baroreceptors, associated with the increased central inspiratory neuronal activity and activity of pulmonary stretch afferents.

In man, the evidence of a carotid chemoreceptor contribution to the cardiovascular responses occurring in breath-hold diving is inevitably more indirect, but the results from several lines of research indicate that the intensity of the diving response can be increased by hypoxia acting via the peripheral chemoreceptors [15].

▶ The diving response is a pattern of responses, consisting of apnoea, bradycardia and selective peripheral vasoconstiction, and can be elicited by stimulation of several difference groups of receptors, sucha s those in the skin of the face, naseal mucosa, pharynx and larynx. It constitutes a defence mechanism against asphyxia and protects the lungs from inhalation of noxious gases and vapours, and vomit.

▶ In breath-hold diving, the response is triggered by excitation of receptors in the skin of the face, and is then reinforced by stimulation of the carotid body chemoreceptors during the progressive asphyxial stage of the dive.

▶ The powerful inhibitory input to respiration from the trigeminal receptors opposes the increasing carotid chemoreceptor drive and suppresses the central inspiratory neurones to the rising level of $PaCO_2$, with the result that the onset in the compelling urge to breathe is delayed.

▶ The appearance of the cardioinhibitory and vasoconstrictor responses is dependent on the occurrence of apnoea through suppression of secondary respiratory mechanisms, the central inspiratory drive and activity of lung stretch afferents.

Medical implications

The respiratory–cardiovascular integrative mechanisms of the types described in this review are important as much for our understanding of the overall control of the cardiovascular system as for their possible role in certain clinical conditions, particularly those associated with periods of apnoea [15,21]. Potentially dangerous situations can arise as a result of apnoea, evoked centrally or reflexly, when the cardiac vagal motoneurones become excessively responsive to excitatory inputs from several groups of receptors (Fig. 11). The result is an exaggerated form of the diving response. Even under laboratory conditions, elicitation of the diving response can lead to profound bradycardia and temporary cardiac arrest in adult animals and to death in the newborn [1]. It must be said that the reflexes arising from the face and upper airways have not received the recognition they deserve, particularly in textbooks of physiology, bearing in mind their potential potency. Even so, forensic scientists have for many years been aware of the importance of reflexly induced vagal mechanisms in the production of cardiac irregularities, bradycardia and arrest of the heart. Cardiac arrest is recognized as a rare but established cause of unconsciousness and death that occurs during submersion when water enters the nose. Indeed, this explanation was put forward as a possible cause of death of three wives of George Joseph Smith in the murder trial held at the Central Criminal Court at the Old Bailey in London, in 1915, known as 'The Case of the Brides in the Bath' [22]. In addition, receptors in the nose of the rabbit can be stimulated by

bronchodilator drugs administered in aerosol form, causing apnoea and temporary cardiac arrest. The active ingredient of the aerosol is the propellant, a mixture of fluorocarbons [1].

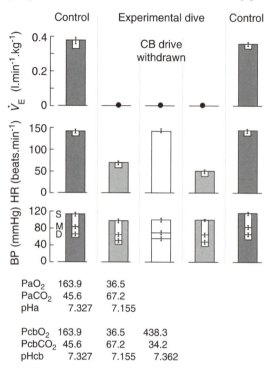

	Control	Experimental dive	Control
PaO_2	163.9	36.5	
$PaCO_2$	45.6	67.2	
pHa	7.327	7.155	
$PcbO_2$	163.9	36.5	438.3
$PcbCO_2$	45.6	67.2	34.2
pHcb	7.327	7.155	7.362

Fig. 10. **The effects of withdrawal of the carotid body chemoreceptor drive on the diving response elicited by face immersion in the seal**

The carotid sinus–carotid body regions on both sides were autoperfused under controlled conditions with blood from a carotid artery. Carotid sinus mean and pulse pressures maintained constant. Dark shaded blocks, control values in spontaneously breathing animals before and after experimental dives; light shaded blocks in second column, values taken 105 s after start of experimental dive; open blocks, withdrawal of chemoreceptor drive during breath-hold dive by perfusion of the carotid bodies with blood of high PO_2 and normal PCO_2 from an external oxygenator; light shaded blocks in fourth column, chemoreceptor drive was re-established during dive by perfusion of the carotid bodies with hypoxic hypercapnic blood from the animal's circulation. Values for PO_2 for arterial blood (a) and blood perfusing the carotid bodies (cb) are expressed in mmHg. Data indicate mean values ± S.E.M. (n = 11). Abbreviations used: $\dot{V}_E$, respiratory minute volume; HR, heart rate; BP, arterial blood pressure (M, mean; S, systolic; D, diastolic). Data taken from [19].

Whether this was the cause of the increase in mortality in asthmatics who used these preparations in the period 1959–1965 is still a matter of conjecture.

Reflexes from the larynx can cause apnoea, profound bradycardia and cardiac arrest in certain circumstances, e.g. during tracheal intubation, extubation, bronchoscopy, laryngoscopy and tracheal suction, unless the vagal postganglionic nerve endings are adequately blocked pharmacologically. Persistent apnoea would lead to excitation of the carotid body chemoreceptors through progressive hypoxaemia and hypercapnia. The paradox of this situation is that, although the excitatory input from the carotid body chemoreceptors to the cardiac vagal motoneurones would enhance the bradycardia, it would not necessarily restart breathing (Figs. 9 and 11). A similar combination of reflexes has been postulated as a cause of death

in some victims of sudden infant death syndrome (SIDS or cot death as it is more commonly known), particularly in those premature and full-term infants prone to episodes of periodic breathing and spells of apnoea [21]. This is supported by the findings that, in human neonates, the peripheral arterial chemoreceptor bradycardia evoked by mild hypoxia is markedly potentiated by apnoea elicited by stimulation of the oropharynx [23], as in laboratory animals [2] (Fig. 6). The combination of impaired or immature central drive to respiration and gastro-oesophageal reflux, which itself causes apnoea, cyanosis and bradycardia, could well trigger such an episode.

The interactions between respiration and the vagal control of heart rate may also be important in the treatment of cardiac irregularities and sinus arrest. In cases of supraventricular paroxysmal tachycardia in adults, the elicita-

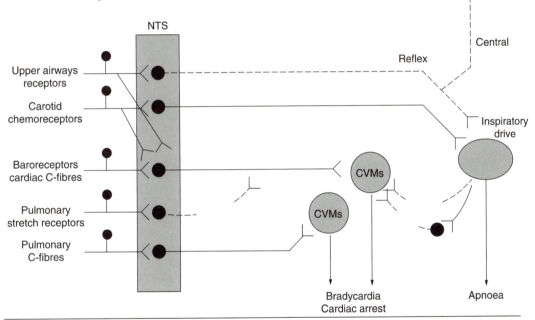

Fig. 11. Diagram illustrating the possible control of the cardiac vagal motoneurones (CVMs) in clinical conditions associated with periodic hypoventilation or apnoea induced centrally or reflexly by stimulation of receptors in the upper airways (e.g. larynx), and with cyanosis causing excitation of the carotid body chemoreceptors

The inhibition of respiration usually occurs in the end-expiratory position and results from cessation of inspiratory neuronal activity and is accompanied by a reduction in the input from pulmonary stretch afferents. This is indicated in the diagram by interruption of the relevant inhibitory pathways to the CVMs. The full expression is now possible of the excitatory inputs to CVMs from upper airways receptors, carotid chemoreceptors, cardiac

C-fibre endings stimulated by increased diastolic volume of the heart, and arterial baroreceptors. The result is a marked bradycardia and even cardiac arrest. The inhibitory effects on the inspiratory neurones are prepotent over the excitatory input resulting from stimulation of the carotid chemoreceptors. Continuous lines, excitatory pathways; dashed lines, inhibitory pathways.

tion of the diving response can be used to revert the heart to normal rhythm where other treatments, such as carotid sinus pressure, have been unsuccessful [24]. The method here is to apply a cold, wet towel to the face of the patient who has been instructed to hold his breath in the end-expiratory position.

It has been shown that an experimentally induced vagal cardiac arrest during an apnoeic episode can be terminated by artificial inflation of the lungs [25]. The restoration of the heart beat is dependent on the innervation to the lungs and is due to disinhibition of the cardiac vagal motoneurones by the activity of pulmonary stretch afferents driven by lung inflation. This mechanism could be invoked in the resuscitation procedures to restore the heart beat in patients with sinus arrest by a few quick inflations of the lungs by the mouth-to-mouth method of artificial respiration. Furthermore, the restoration of the heart beat in a patient with sinus bradycardia, or arrest resulting from coronary angiography, can often be achieved by asking him to take a deep breath or to cough. The mechanism involved may be a combination of a central inspiratory neuronal drive and activity of pulmonary stretch afferents causing refractoriness of the cardiac vagal motoneurones to the excitatory input from cardiac C-fibres (Fig. 11).

▶ In certain clinical conditions, associated with episodes of apnoea combined with asphyxia, a patient could be at risk of severe bradycardia or cardiac arrest.
▶ During episodes of apnoea, the cardiac vagal motoneurones become maximally responsive to excitatory inputs from several groups of cardiovascular receptors, such as arterial baroreceptors and chemoreceptors, and upper airway receptors.
▶ Stimulation of one or more of these inputs would, under these conditions, lead to bradycardia and cardiac arrest.
▶ Clinical conditions in which patients are at risk of cardiac arrest are discussed. The same combination of mechanisms could be responsible, in some cases at least, for the sudden infant death syndrome.
▶ A vagally induced arrested heart during apnoea can be restarted by inflation of the lungs through disinhibition of the cardiac vagal motoneurones, as a result of excitation of lung stretch afferents.

Conclusion

▶ Mechanisms involved in the integration of the respiratory and cardiovascular control systems play an important role in the control of the circulation by inputs from peripheral vascular receptors.
▶ Under circumstances in which respiration is increased, the primary cardiac and vascular responses to stimulation of the carotid body chemoreceptors, bradycardia and vasoconstriction, respectively, are partly or wholly suppressed, or even reversed.
▶ The full expression of the primary responses can only be seen when respiration is inhibited, either centrally or reflexly.
▶ The mechanisms by which respiration affects the excitatory input from the chemo-receptors include changes in the central inspiratory neuronal drive, changes in activity of slowly adapting pulmonary stretch receptors and alterations in $PaCO_2$.
▶ These integrative mechanisms which are involved in overall control of the cardiovascular system are important in conditions such as systemic hypoxia, hypocapnia, haemorrhagic hypotension, and apnoeic asphyxia [1,2], in addition to breath-hold diving [14].
▶ It follows that, in studies of the evaluation of the action of drugs on the cardiovascular system in the intact organism, the observed responses may, in part at least, be determined by any concomitant changes in pulmonary ventilation through the modification of cardiovascular reflexes and the direct effects of changes in blood gases on peripheral blood vessels. Investigations of this sort, although they may be primarily directed towards actions on the cardiovascular system, should therefore include measurements of respiratory variables and/or activity in a phrenic nerve and arterial blood gases to enable a full analysis to be made of the mechanisms involved.

References

(References [1–15] are essential reading.)

1. Daly, M. de B. (1986) Interactions between respiration and circulation. In Handbook of Physiology, Section III, Volume 2, Part II (Cherniack, N.S. and Widdicombe, J.G., eds.), pp. 529–594, Am. Physiol. Soc., Bethesda

2. Daly, M. de B. (1983) Peripheral arterial chemoreceptors and the cardiovascular system. In Physiology of the Peripheral Arterial Chemoreceptors (Acker, H. and O'Regan, R.G., eds.), pp. 325–393, Elsevier, Amsterdam

3. Widdicombe, J.G. (1981) Nervous receptors in the respiratory tract and lungs. In Regulation of Breathing (Hornbein, T.F., ed.), Series, Lung Biology in Health and Disease, Volume 17. pp. 429-472. Marcel Dekker, New York

4. Coleridge, H.M. and Coleridge, J.C.G. (1986) Reflexes evoked from tracheobronchial tree and lungs. In Handbook of Physiology, Section 3, Volume 2, Part I (Cherniack, N.S. and Widdicombe, J.G., eds.), pp. 395–429, Am. Physiol. Soc., Bethesda

5. von Euler, C. (1986) Brain stem mechanisms for generation and control of breathing pattern. In Handbook of Physiology, Section III, Volume 2, Part I (Cherniack, N.S. and Widdicombe, J.G., eds.), pp. 1–67, Am. Physiol. Soc., Bethesda

6. Spyer, K.M. (1984) Central control of the cardiovascular system. In Recent Advances in Physiology (Baker, P.F., ed.), pp. 163–200, Churchill Livingstone, Edinburgh

7. Jordan, D. and Spyer, K.M. (1987) Central neural mechanisms mediating respiratory–cardiovascular interactions. In Neurobiology of the Cardiorespiratory System (Taylor, E.W., ed.), pp. 322–341, Manchester University Press, Manchester

8. Loewy, A.D. (1990) Central autonomic pathways. In Central Regulation of Autonomic Functions (Loewy, A.D. and Spyer, K.M., eds), pp. 88–103, Oxford University Press, Oxford

9. Loewy, A.D. and Spyer, K.M. (1990) Vagal preganglionic neurones. In Central Regulation of Autonomic Functions (Loewy, A.D. and Spyer, K.M., eds.), pp. 68–87, Oxford University Press, Oxford

10. Spyer, K.M. (1990) The central organisation of reflex circulatory control. In Central Regulation of Autonomic Functions (Loewy, A.D. and Spyer, K.M., eds.), pp. 168–188, Oxford University Press, Oxford

11. Coote, J.H. (1988) The organisation of cardiovascular neurons in the spinal cord. Rev. Physiol. Biochem. Pharmacol. 110, 148–285

12. Guyenet, P.G. (1990) Role of ventral medulla oblongata in blood pressure regulation. In Central Regulation of Autonomic Functions (Loewy, A.D. and Spyer, K.M., eds.), pp. 145–167, Oxford University Press, Oxford

13. Heymans, C. and Neil, E. (1958) Reflexogenic Areas of the Cardiovascular System, Churchill, London

14. Daly, M. de B. (1984) Breath-hold diving: mechanisms of cardiovascular adjustments in the mammal. In Recent Advances in Physiology (Baker, P.F., ed.), pp. 201–245, Churchill Livingstone, Edinburgh

15. Elsner, R. and Gooden, B.A. (1983) Diving and Asphyxia, Cambridge University Press, Cambridge

16. Haymet, B.T. and McCloskey, D.I. (1975) Baroreceptor and chemoreceptor influences on heart rate during the respiratory cycle in the dog. J. Physiol. 246, 699–712

17. Angell-James, J.E. and Daly, M. de B. (1975) Some aspects of upper respiratory tract reflexes. Acta Oto-Laryngol. 79, 242–251

18. Black, A.M.S. and Torrance, R.W. (1971) Respiratory oscillations in chemoreceptor discharge in the control of breathing. Resp. Physiol. 13, 221–237

19. Daly, M. de B., Elsner, R. and Angell-James, J.E. (1977) Cardio-respiratory control by the carotid chemoreceptors during experimental dives in the seal. Am. J. Physiol. 232, H508–H516

20. Angell-James, J.E., Daly, M. de B. and Elsner, R. (1978) Arterial baroreceptor reflexes in the seal and their modification during experimental dives. Am. J. Physiol. 234, H730–H739

21. Daly, M. de B., Angell-James, J.E. and Elsner, R. (1979) Role of carotid-body chemoreceptors and their reflex interactions in bradycardia and cardiac arrest. Lancet i, 764–767

22. Angell-James, J.E. and Daly, M. de B. (1969) Nasal reflexes. Proc. R. Soc. Med. 62, 1287–1293

23. Wennergren, G., Hertzberg, T., Milerad, J., Bjure, J. and Lagercrantz, H. (1989) Hypoxia reinforces laryngeal reflex bradycardia in infants. Acta Paediat. Scand. 78, 11–17

24. Wildenthal, K. and Atkins, J.M. (1979) Use of the 'diving reflex' for the treatment of paroxysmal supraventricular tachycardia. Am. Heart J. 98, 536–537

25. Angell-James, J.E. and Daly, M. de B. (1978) The effects of artificial lung inflation on reflexly induced bradycardia associated with apnoea in the dog. J. Physiol. 274, 349–366

26. Daly, M. de B. and Kirkman, E. (1988) Cardiovascular responses to stimulation of pulmonary C fibres in the cat: their modulation by changes in respiration. J. Physiol. 402, 43–63

27. Daly, M. de B. and Angell-James, J.E. (1979) The 'diving response' and its possible clinical implications. Int. Med. 1, 12–19

3

Cardiovascular changes associated with behavioural alerting

Janice M. Marshall

Department of Physiology, The Medical School, Birmingham B15 2TT, U.K.

Introduction

The ability to show behavioural alerting in response to unexpected or noxious environmental stimuli, and to show defensive or aggressive behaviour if the stimulus is sufficiently strong, would seem to be essential for the survival of the individual and of the species. On the other hand, since all mammals generally spend part of every 24 hours asleep, it would seem that sleep too is essential for survival. These two very different patterns of behaviour are accompanied by different patterns of cardiovascular response, which in some ways contrast directly with one another. The purpose of this and the following chapter is to discuss these cardiovascular patterns, to consider their underlying neural mechanisms and their functional significance.

The alerting response

The alerting or defence response? An historical perspective

It was Cannon (1929) who gave the earliest accounts of the bodily changes that occur in what he called 'emergency' reactions [1]. Studies on the cat led him to conclude that there is an increase in arterial pressure, tachycardia and a diversion of blood from the viscera and skin towards muscle, due to vasoconstriction in the former and vasodilatation in the latter. Cannon recognized this pattern as one which would best prepare the animal for the muscular exertion that was likely to follow. From venous blood samples, taken from the cat during aggressive behaviour and assayed on uterine and intestinal muscle *in vitro*, Cannon deduced that adrenin (adrenaline) was largely responsi-ble for these changes, although he acknowl-edged that differential changes in the sympa-thetic nerve activity to the tissues probably sup-ported the actions of the hormone. To put this into context, relatively little was known about the autonomic nervous system at the time.

The work of Bard, who began his research as Cannon's student, was important in indicat-ing the parts of the brain that are concerned with emotional behaviour. Bard and colleagues found that cats that had been decerebrated at the collicular level were able to display 'sham rage' in response to even very mild tactile stim-uli. However, they discovered that for the behavioural response to be well-organized and of normal intensity, relative to that seen in the cat with intact brain, it was essential that the level of decerebration preserved the hypothala-mus. This led to the idea that, while parts of the midbrain may be important in aggressive behaviour, the hypothalamus was in some way a key co-ordinating centre.

Later, studies of Hess and collaborators, for which Hess won the Nobel prize, took the field a major step forward, for they began to identify (by localized electrical stimulation) the regions of the brain concerned with specific patterns of behaviour. Again, they identified the hypothalamus as a region of major impor-tance in aggressive behaviour, but within the hypothalamus they singled out a region lying posteriorly and medial, ventral and lateral to the fornix (see Fig. 6, later). Mild electrical stimula-tion in this region evoked alerting behaviour, while stronger stimulation led to fight or attack. It was at this stage that the term defence reac-tion (Abweh reaktion) was coined to describe all types of affective behaviour [1].

After this, Swedish workers led by Folkow and Oberg [2] began to investigate a group of sympathetic dilator fibres that supply skeletal muscle of cats and dogs and which seemed unusual in that they used acetylcholine as a transmitter and were not involved in homeostatic reflexes. By using electrical stimulation they traced a 'dilator' pathway through the hypothalamus, midbrain and medulla and found that it ran through the hypothalamic region identified by Hess and colleagues. They also noted that when electrical stimulation evoked vasodilatation in muscle, this was commonly accompanied by cutaneous and splanchnic vasoconstriction.

The significance of the association of the behavioural and cardiovascular components of affective behaviour in the same locations in the brain was first emphasized by Abrahams, Hilton and Zbrozyna [1]. In a series of experiments on the cat in the early 1960s, they showed conclusively that the area from which muscle vasodilatation, tachycardia, cutaneous and splanchnic vasoconstriction could be evoked in the anaesthetized cat (Figs. 1 and 2) was the same area from which behavioural alerting, culminating in flight or defensive behaviour, could be evoked in the conscious cat. Indeed, even in the anaesthetized animal, pupillary dilatation, retraction of the nictitating membrane and piloerection accompanied the cardiovascular response, just as they accompa-

nied the behavioural response in the conscious state. Since in the conscious cat the characteristic pattern of cardiovascular response was apparent, even when the animal showed only pupillary dilatation and pricking of the ears and before it showed obvious aggressive behaviour, Abrahams, Hilton and Zbrozyna always referred to the cardiovascular response as being characteristic of 'the alerting stage of the defence reaction'. Indeed, they echoed Cannon's proposal (see above) that a redistribution of blood flow — away from viscera and towards muscle — would serve as a preparation for muscular exertion. However, probably because the phrase 'alerting stage of the defence reaction' is cumbersome, many who have since worked on this cardiovascular response have referred to it simply as the defence response. This is regrettable because the cardiovascular pattern has become associated with aggressive behaviour, rather than with the more everyday occurrence of behavioural alerting.

The full pattern of response
Putting together the results of many different studies, it is clear that the pattern of splanchnic, renal and cutaneous vasoconstriction, vasodilatation in skeletal muscle and tachycardia is accompanied by an increase in cardiac contractility, venoconstriction and an increase in

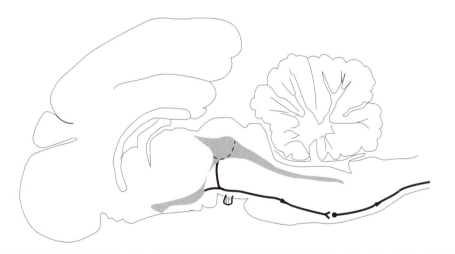

Fig. I. **Diagrammatic sagittal section of cat's brain**
Hatched areas represent regions in hypothalamus, midbrain and medulla from which the pattern of the alerting response can be evoked by electrical stimulation; solid line indicates location of efferent pathway for cardiovascular pattern of response and other autonomic components. Reproduced with permission from [1].

cardiac output. The mobilization of blood reservoirs may be supported by a decrease in pulmonary vascular compliance, while the concomitant tachypnoea and hyperpnoea may improve pulmonary gas exchange. In addition, there is evidence that skeletal muscle fatigues more slowly during maintained contraction, an effect which was first described by Cannon, but has since been elaborated by several groups [1,2].

A purist might argue that all of these components should be recorded together for a response evoked by a particular stimulus to be regarded as that of the alerting stage of the defence reaction; this is seldom practical. However, given that a variety of stimuli can evoke generalized vasodilatation (not only in skeletal muscle, but in other tissues as well) and that a variety of stimuli can evoke generalized vasoconstriction, it is most important that muscle vasodilatation and splanchnic vasoconstriction be recorded together, or, at the very least, that muscle vasodilatation be recorded simultaneously with a rise in arterial pressure. It should also be shown that the muscle vasodilatation is a primary rather than a secondary response to hyperventilation (see Chapter 2) or muscle contraction (see Chapter 7), while the simple observation that the cardiovascular response is accompanied by pupillary dilatation would provide supportive evidence.

A response pattern that accompanies behavioural alerting

The experiments on conscious cats showed that localized electrical stimulation in the brain could evoke muscle vasodilatation in the absence of muscle contraction, and that this could be accompanied by alerting behaviour without any sign of aggressive or defensive behaviour. They also showed that the same was true when a sudden auditory stimulus, or a mild painful stimulus, was applied. Experiments performed by Caraffa-Braga and colleagues allowed a more complete analysis [3]. They found that when a dog was startled by the noise of two saucepan lids being rattled together, it would turn towards the sound showing no sign of aggression, but there was a prompt tachycardia, splanchnic and renal vasoconstriction, vasodilatation in hindlimb muscle and usually a rise in arterial pressure. When the behavioural response produced by this or other stimuli, such as the firing of a pistol or ice water being

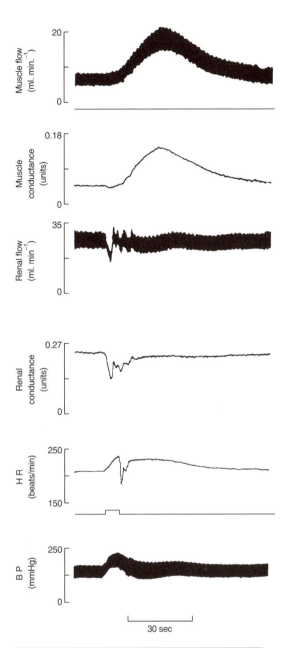

Fig. 2. The cardiovascular pattern of the alerting response evoked in the anaesthetized cat by electrical stimulation in the brainstem defence areas

Abbreviations used: BP, arterial blood pressure; HR, heart rate. Renal and muscle conductance were calculated as renal and muscle blood flow/arterial blood pressure. The period of stimulation is indicated by the bar below the heart-rate trace. Reproduced with permission from R.J. Timms.

squirted into the face, was more intense, then the cardiovascular changes became more pronounced. However, even when the animal simply changed from the resting state lying down, to alertness, with head raised and ears pricked, there was slight splanchnic and renal vasoconstriction, muscle vasodilatation and tachycardia, the balance of these haemodynamic effects often leading to a fall in arterial pressure.

One could question whether humans respond like other mammals for human subjects cajoled into performing difficult mental arithmetic to the beat of a metronome, or subjected to a cold pressor test (putting one hand or foot into ice-cold water) may show signs of embarrassment or anxiety, but rarely aggression. However, under such circumstances, they too show the characteristic pattern of an increase in cardiac output, renal and cutaneous vasoconstriction and vasodilatation in limb muscle in the absence of limb movement [4] (Fig. 4).

In fact, the simplest conclusion to draw is that just as the behavioural response evoked by

a novel, noxious or emotionally stressful stimulus can be graded from increased alertness, to orienting to the site of the stimulus, to frank aggressive or defensive behaviour, so too can the accompanying pattern of cardiovascular response (see Table 1). It seems that vasodilatation in skeletal muscle is the most readily evoked component, while a rise in arterial pressure occurs when the increase in cardiac output and vasoconstrictor components is strong enough to overcome the muscle vasodilatation.

Species distribution
It is apparent from the studies referred to above that the cardiovascular components of the alerting response can be readily evoked by environmental stimuli in the cat, dog and man. They have also been evoked in the monkey by electrical stimulation in the hypothalamus and in the baboon by a natural environmental stimulus, such as confrontation with a snake. Further, in both the rat and rabbit under anaesthesia, the full cardiovascular response can be evoked by localized electrical stimulation in the brain,

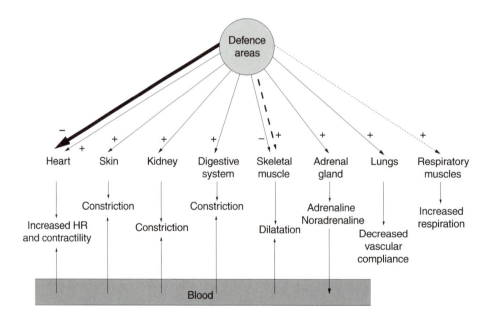

Fig. 3. **Schematic diagram indicating the respiratory and cardiovascular components of the alerting response and the changes in nerve activity that produce them**

In the upper part of the figure thin solid lines indicate influences on sympathetic noradrenergic outflow; thick solid line indicates influence on parasympathetic outflow; thick dashed line indicates influence on sympathetic cholinergic outflow; thin dotted line indicates influence on somatic motor outflow; + and − indicate increase and decrease in activity, respectively.

while in the conscious state stimulation at these same sites evoked alerting, culminating in aggressive behaviour. Few would doubt that the rat shows alerting or aggressive behaviour in the wild, but the rabbit might be thought of as a placid animal. However, rabbits in the wild do show behavioural alerting when startled, and strong aggression when defending territory or competing for a female. Even the opossum, which is well-known for its 'playing dead' behaviour, can show the cardiovascular pattern of the alerting response upon electrical stimulation in the brain, at least under anaesthesia.

In the light of such evidence, it seems a reasonable hypothesis that all mammals have the neural substrate required to produce the cardiovascular components of the alerting response.

▶ Unexpected, novel or noxious stimuli can evoke behavioural alerting, culminating in aggressive or defensive behaviour if the stimulus is sufficiently strong. This is accompanied by a characteristic pattern of cardiovascular response whose magnitude is graded with stimulus intensity. It includes an increase in cardiac output and a redistribution of blood flow away from skin, gastrointestinal tract and kidney, towards skeletal muscle, due to vasoconstriction and vasodilatation, respectively.

▶ The increase in muscle blood flow is promoted by an accompanying rise in arterial pressure which is itself facilitated when the stimulus is strong by central suppression of the baroreceptor reflex. This response pattern can be conditioned in the classic Pavlovian manner. Its individual components show habituation or sensitization when the stimulus is repeated.

The mediation of the efferent pattern of response

Pharmacological and neurophysiological evidence indicates that the cardiac components of the response are mediated by a decrease in parasympathetic activity and an increase in sympathetic activity, while the splanchnic, renal and cutaneous vasoconstriction and the venoconstriction are due to increased sympathetic noradrenergic activity (Fig. 3).

It is probably muscle vasodilatation that has attracted the greatest interest (Table 1). The early work of Folkow and co-workers demonstrated that, in the cat and dog, the dilatation is mainly mediated by activation of sympathetic cholinergic fibres [2]. This has been confirmed many times; however, there is evidence, at least in the cat, that inhibition of the activity of sympathetic noradrenergic fibre activity and the effect of circulating adrenaline on β-adrenoreceptors contribute to the muscle vasodilatation, possibly to varying degrees in different animals.

There is no histochemical or pharmacological evidence of a sympathetic cholinergic supply to skeletal muscle in either the rat or rabbit. In the rat, the dilatation may be wholly explained by the combined effect of a decrease in sympathetic noradrenergic activity and circulating catecholamines [5]. However, in the rabbit, neither of these mechanisms provides an adequate explanation, nor could the dilatation be blocked by histamine antagonists. Instead, it has been attributed to activation of purinergic fibres that release ATP as a transmitter [6].

The situation in non-human primates is relatively clear. Histochemical studies failed to demonstrate a sympathetic cholinergic supply to muscle in the monkey (*Macaca iris*), and stimulation of the sympathetic chain after blockade of the sympathetic noradrenergic fibres evoked no response in muscle in four different species of monkey, or in the baboon. In addition, the muscle vasodilatation evoked in the squirrel monkey by electrical stimulation in the hypothalamic defence area was insensitive to atropine. On the other hand, the muscle vasodilatation produced in the conscious baboon as part of the alerting response was blocked by propranolol, indicating that it was mediated by circulating adrenaline.

As far as man is concerned, it is widely stated in standard textbooks that the muscle vasodilatation that occurs in acute emotional stress is mediated by cholinergic fibres. However, histochemical studies performed on biopsy material from human muscles failed to show any cholinergic supply to the blood vessels. Further, neurophysiological recordings from the nerve supply to muscle of human subjects has failed to demonstrate fibres with characteristics similar to those of cholinergic fibres in the cat, i.e. there were no fibres whose activity lacked baroreceptor modulation, but which were activated during emotional stress.

Table 1. **Vasodilatation in skeletal muscle**

Species	Decrease in noradrenergic activity	Increase in cholinergic activity	Other nerve fibres	Increase in circulating catecholamines
Cat	+	+	?	+
Dog	+	+	?	+
Rat	+	0	?	+
Rabbit	+	0	+	+
Man	+	?	?	+

The oft-quoted idea that the increase in forearm blood flow that occurs during emotional stress is mediated by activation of dilator fibres, was based on the finding that the response produced by mental arithmetic was somewhat reduced by acute sympathetic blockade [7]. Cholinergic fibres were implicated because the increase in blood flow was judged to be smaller after intra-arterial injection of

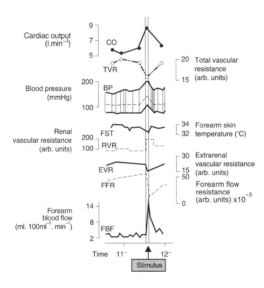

Fig. 4. The pattern of response evoked in a human subject by mental arithmetic

Total vascular (peripheral) resistance was calculated as cardiac output/arterial blood pressure. Skin temperature was used as an indication of skin blood flow. Extrarenal vascular resistance includes the total vascular resistance of peripheral tissues other than that of the kidneys. Forearm flow resistance was calculated as arterial blood pressure/forearm blood flow. Reproduced with permission from [3].

atropine into the forearm. However, this evidence was rather inconclusive. First, the increase in forearm blood flow evoked in individual subjects after acute sympathetic blockade, or after administration of atropine, was at most 25–30% smaller than before, and in some subjects it was larger than before. This variability was no greater than that seen in the response to mental arithmetic before either sympathetic blockade or atropine injection. Secondly, such small differences in the blood flow changes could well have been accounted for by differences in the changes in arterial pressure evoked by mental arithmetic, rather than by differences in the changes in forearm vascular resistance; this possibility could not be assessed, since arterial pressure was not recorded.

On the other hand, the fact that a substantial increase in forearm blood flow occurred in response to mental arithmetic, even after local sympathetic blockade, suggests that vasodilatation was at least partly mediated by hormones. The observation that its magnitude and time-course could be mimicked in normal subjects by intravenous infusion of adrenaline, and that it was virtually absent in patients who had been adrenalectomized, strongly implicated adrenaline as the mediator. Thus the simplest conclusion would be that, in this respect, man is like other primates. The possibility that there are dilator fibres to muscles that use a transmitter other than acetylcholine awaits investigation (see Chapter 7).

If, as has been generally supposed, sympathetic cholinergic fibres are activated only during the alerting stage of the defence response, then the fact that stimulation of the sympathetic chain after noradrenergic blockade could evoke atropine-sensitive muscle dilatation in the sheep, goat and fox, indicates that in these species the muscle vasodilatation of the alerting response is at least partly cholinergic. However, since under the same experimental conditions stimulation of the sympathetic chain failed to evoke muscle vasodilatation in the pole cat, badger, opossum, rat or hare, it can be presumed that other mediators are responsible in these species [2].

> ▶ The cardiovascular pattern of the alerting response is mediated by a patterned change in autonomic activity: a decrease in parasympathetic and increase in sympathetic activity to the heart, and an increase in sympathetic activity to splanchnic, renal and cutaneous circulations and to venous vessels.
> ▶ The vasodilatation in skeletal muscle is probably produced by a decrease in sympathetic noradrenergic activity to muscle, by circulating adrenaline and by activation of sympathetic cholinergic or other dilator fibres.
> ▶ Overall, the alerting response ensures that an increased cardiac output is preferentially distributed to skeletal muscle at high arterial perfusion pressure.

The appropriate stimulus

Experiments carried out on a range of unanaesthetized mammals and on human subjects indicate that the full pattern of the alerting response can be produced by a variety of novel or unexpected stimuli, and by stimuli that portend threat or danger, or create emotional stress. Sudden auditory stimuli have proved effective in a variety of species, including man, as has pain in the form of mild electrical stimuli applied to the skin, or the cold pressor test. To some extent, the appropriate stimuli are species specific. Thus, the sight of a dog may be enough to evoke the full cardiovascular response in a cat, but would be unlikely to have the same effect in most members of the human species. On the other hand, the sight of an examination hall, the bank manager, or the dentist might be very effective in the average student, but would be of little significance, and therefore have little cardiovascular effect, in the average cat.

It is also clear that a stimulus which has no significance the first time it occurs, can acquire significance and produce the pattern of the alerting response if it is coupled with a stimulus that does have significance as a potential threat.

In other words, the alerting response can be conditioned [1,2]. An everyday example of this would be the child who goes to the dentist for the first time: if the child has no older brother or sister to tell him/her what can happen in a dental surgery, he/she is unlikely to show any cardiovascular response before entering the surgery. However, if he/she has an unpleasant experience during that first visit, then on the second visit the mere sight of the waiting room may be enough to evoke the full response. Such conditioning has been demonstrated in experimental studies on dogs, cats and baboons when the response to the noxious stimulus applied to the skin, or to running on a treadmill, has been conditioned to presentation of a coloured light, or a sound.

Many years ago, the work on anaesthetized animals established that the cardiovascular components of the alerting response cannot be evoked by stimulation of afferent inputs in animals that are anaesthetized with the commonly used anaesthetics, such as chloralose, urethane, barbiturates and halothane. This indicates that such anaesthetics block synaptic inputs into the brainstem defence areas. On the other hand, cats decerebrated at the thalamic level, so as to remove all cortical structures but leaving the hypothalamus and brainstem intact (see above), do not require anaesthesia and, in such preparations, 'sham rage' [accompanied by a rise in arterial pressure, tachycardia and muscle vasodilatation that was not secondary to muscle contraction (see Chapter 7)] could readily be evoked, not only by physical stimuli that would be effective in the conscious animal, but by selective stimulation of the carotid chemoreceptors. This indicated that carotid chemoreceptors can provide an excitatory input to the defence areas, albeit when cortical inhibitory influences are removed.

It became possible to investigate this more fully when it was discovered that the steroid anaesthetic alphaxolone–alphadalone (Althesin or Saffan) can be used at a dose which produces full anaesthesia, but does not block afferent inputs to the defence areas to the same extent as other anaesthetics [8]. In cats or rats anaesthetized with Althesin or Saffan, selective stimulation of the carotid chemoreceptors could evoke the full cardiovascular pattern of the alerting response accompanied by the other autonomic signs of alerting which are characteristic to these species. Thus, when the chemoreceptor stimulus was strong, as judged by the magnitude of the respiratory response, the pattern of the alerting response completely overcame the primary bradycardia and generalized vasoconstriction that is evoked by peripheral chemoreceptor stimulation under more conventional anaesthetics. Importantly, it was established that the tachycardia and muscle vasodilatation evoked by strong chemoreceptor stimulation were true primary effects of chemoreceptor stimulation and not secondary to hyperventilation or muscle contraction [9].

Following this, it was found that in cats and rats anaesthetized with Saffan, acute systemic hypoxia which reduced arterial oxygen pressure (PaO_2) to 58 mmHg or below could also produce the full cardiovascular pattern of the alerting response. Moreover, in conscious rats, exposure to hypoxia induced short periods of behavioural alerting that were accompanied by tachycardia and raised arterial pressure [10]. These observations suggest that systemic hypoxia can serve as an alerting stimulus in the same way as auditory or painful stimuli. This is fully consistent with the many reports that acute systemic hypoxia produces behavioural arousal in a variety of different species, including man.

Since the pattern of the alerting response can be produced by a variety of different stimuli, it seems probable that a stimulus of one modality, which is of insufficient strength by itself to evoke a recognizable response, may nevertheless raise the level of activity in the defence areas sufficiently to lower the threshold for a stimulus of a different modality. For example, a sub-threshold level of hypoxia experienced by a rat in a sewer may lower the threshold for an auditory stimulus to produce the full response, while acute emotional stress produced in a human subject by an asthmatic attack might lower the threshold for systemic hypoxia to produce the full response.

> ▶ The alerting response can be evoked by a wide variety of stimuli ranging from sudden sound, to peripheral chemoreceptor stimulation, to acute pain.
> ▶ Some stimuli are species specific.
> ▶ The alerting response can be conditioned in the classic Pavlovian manner.

Inhibition of the baroreceptor reflex

The fact that the pattern of response evoked by electrical stimulation within the hypothalamic defence area included a rise in arterial pressure and a simultaneous tachycardia raised the possibility that the baroreceptor reflex was inhibited. Indeed, it was demonstrated in the 1960s that during such a response the reflex bradycardia and fall in arterial pressure that can normally be evoked by raising the pressure in a vascularly isolated preparation of the carotid sinus did not occur. Thus it was proposed that both the cardiac and vascular components of the baroreceptor reflex are inhibited during activation of the defence areas [1].

While there has been general acceptance, from similar studies involving electrical stimulation in the hypothalamus, that the cardiac component of the baroreceptor reflex is suppressed, there has been controversy over the vascular component. Notably, it was argued that the baroreceptor-mediated reflex dilatation is not only preserved, but that it is very important because it augments the muscle vasodilatation of the alerting response, limits the splanchnic vasoconstriction, and thereby reduces the work-load of the heart by reducing after-load. This idea has an immediate attraction; however, when it was tested in a study on 32 cats, the results from only eight of them supported the hypothesis [11].

On the other hand, it was shown in other experiments that electrical stimulation within a localized region of the hypothalamus produced the full cardiovascular pattern of the alerting response and totally inhibited the decrease in cardiac and renal sympathetic nerve activity that was evoked by concurrent baroreceptor stimulation. Nevertheless, stimulation at various sites in the surrounding area often produced some, but not all, components of the alerting response and inhibited the bradycardia. The renal sympathetic component of the baroreceptor reflex was not reduced [12]. Since stimulation at such sites generally evoked an increase in respiration, it seems likely that the inhibition of the cardiac component of the baroreceptor reflex evoked from these sites reflected the strong inhibitory influence of increased central inspiratory drive upon cardiac vagal neurones (see Chapter 2). The implication of this idea is that those who reported inhibition of only the cardiac component, did not

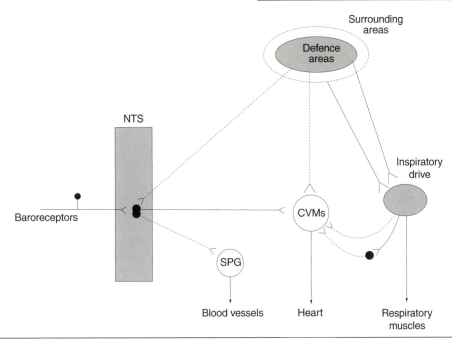

Fig. 5. **Schematic diagram indicating how activation of the defence areas and surrounding areas may modify the baroreceptor reflex**
Abbreviations used: NTS, nucleus tractus solitarius; SPG, sympathetic preganglionic neurones; CVM, cardiac vagal motoneurones. Continuous lines indicate excitatory influence; dotted lines indicate inhibitory influence.

stimulate within the defence area proper (Fig. 5).

It should be possible to circumvent the problems encountered in interpreting the effects of electrical stimulation in the brain if the alerting response is evoked as a reflex. When such experiments were performed on cats anaesthetized with Althesin, it was found that if the cardiovascular components of the alerting response were evoked — by electrical stimulation of the radial nerve with parameters chosen to activate the small myelinated and unmyelinated pain fibres, or by stimulation of the carotid chemoreceptors — then the evoked tachycardia, renal vasoconstriction and muscle vasodilatation were unaffected by simultaneous stimulation of carotid baroreceptors. However, during less-intense activation of the defence areas, as judged by the magnitude of the muscle vasodilatation and tachycardia evoked by radial nerve or chemoreceptor stimulation, this pattern of response simply showed algebraic summation with the bradycardia, renal and muscle vasodilatation evoked by baroreceptor stimulation. This led to the suggestion that the degree of inhibition of the cardiac and vascular compo-

nents of the baroreceptor reflex may be graded with the level of activity in the defence areas [9]. This was given some support by the observation that naturally evoked increases in the level of alertness in the unanaesthetized cat were associated with graded suppression of the baroreceptor reflex.

The fact that both the cardiac and vascular components of the baroreceptor reflex can be inhibited during defence area activation is fully consistent with neurophysiological evidence that electrical stimulation in the hypothalamic defence area inhibits neurones within the nucleus tractus solitarius which are activated by baroreceptor stimulation (see Chapter 1).

▶ The arterial baroreceptor reflex is suppressed during the alerting response, probably to an extent that is graded with the magnitude of the alerting response.
▶ During a pronounced alerting response, the cardiac and vascular components of the baroreceptor reflex are completely suppressed.

Central neural organization

Evidence from electrical stimulation

Studies involving localized electrical stimulation within the brain of anaesthetized cats have shown that the full cardiovascular components of the alerting response can be evoked from sites that lie within a strip which runs just rostral and dorsal to the optic chiasma, through the hypothalamus, medial and central to the fornix, to a region just dorsal and lateral to the mamillary bodies and extending laterally as a band which seems to end over the middle of the optic tract [1] (Fig. 6). Throughout the hypothalamus, the location of the effective stimulation sites seems to bear no relationship to any anatomical nuclei. In the midbrain, the cardiovascular pattern could be evoked from the dorsolateral part of the periaqueductal grey matter and from the tegmentum, ventral to the superior colliculus. This region seems to extend as a strip through the dorsal pons to the dorsal medulla, where it finally ends close to the floor of the fourth ventricle in the region that was termed the pressor area of the vasomotor centre (see Chapter 1). Although the cardiovascular pattern elicited from all of these sites was essentially the same, the muscle vasodilatation evoked from the dorsal medullary area was not sensitive to atropine, but was attributed to inhibition of sympathetic noradrenergic activity to muscle [1]. In the conscious cat, electrical stimulation within any of these regions evoked behavioural alerting through to characteristic fight or flight patterns, depending upon the strength of the stimulus.

From comparable studies carried out on the dog, rat, rabbit, opossum, monkey and baboon, it seems that the cardiovascular and behavioural components of the alerting response can be evoked from homologous regions in these species. There is limited information on the effects of electrical stimulation in human subjects; however, the fact that restlessness, anxiety and rage have been evoked from the medial and posterior hypothalamus suggests that the regions are comparable in man.

It has been deduced that the efferent pathway from these defence regions runs from the mamillary bodies, dorsal to the cerebral peduncles, through to the midbrain and then through the ventral medulla, via a route which is dorsal and lateral to the trapezoid bodies and corticospinal tracts (Figs. 1 and 6).

In the conscious cat, alerting and defensive behaviour accompanied by the cardiovascular pattern of the alerting response could also be evoked, by electrical stimulation in a band over the most lateral points of the optic tract and extending through to the basal and central nuclei of the amygdala. The responses evoked from here took longer to develop and were longer-lasting than those evoked from the hypothalamus and more-closely resembled responses evoked by natural stimuli. Lesion experiments demonstrated that the amygdaloid

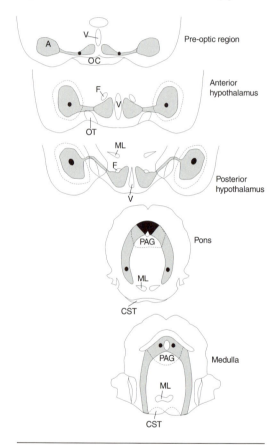

Fig. 6. **Simplified anatomical diagrams of transverse sections of the brain showing the regions from which the alerting response can be evoked by electrical stimulation (grey areas), and by chemical stimulation (black areas)**

Abbreviations used: A, amygdala; CST, corticospinal tract; F, fornix; ML, medial lemniscus; OC, optic chiasma; OT, optic tract; PAG, periaqueductal grey; V, ventricle. Note: not all of the regions identified by electrical stimulation have been explored by chemical stimulation (see text).

defence area is afferent to the hypothalamus, via a pathway over the optic tract. However, the hypothalamic defence area is also afferent to the amygdala, via a pathway which runs through the stria terminalis. This loop, from the amygdala to the hypothalamus and back to the amygdala, may allow a 'reverberating' circuit to develop. This may explain why, once initiated, the alerting response tends to outlast the stimulus.

Since, in cats anaesthetized with commonly used anaesthetics, the cardiovascular pattern of the alerting response could not be evoked from the sites in the amygdala or in the amygdalofugal pathway on the lateral edge of the optic tract, this led to the suggestion that there are important synapses in this region that are especially sensitive to anaesthesia. The fact that in cats anaesthetized with Althesin the full cardiovascular response can be evoked from these very sites emphasizes how useful this anaesthetic can be in studies of central organization of the alerting response.

The motor cortex
Investigations on the route of the central neural pathway that activates the sympathetic cholinergic supply to skeletal muscle in the cat led to the conclusion that cholinergically mediated dilatation could be evoked by electrical stimulation in the motor cortex [2]. It was, therefore, deduced that a pathway from the motor cortex synapses in the hypothalamus and midbrain defence areas, and that this pathway is responsible for increasing the blood flow to muscle before the onset of exercise.

Although this idea appears in the standard textbooks, it was questioned by later studies on the cat which showed that the muscle vasodilatation evoked by electrical stimulation in the motor cortex was always tightly coupled with contraction of that muscle, as judged from electromyogram recordings [13]. The vasodilatation and the muscle contractions had the same thresholds, the magnitudes of the two responses were directly related and procedures which attenuated the muscle contraction caused a parallel reduction in the vasodilatation. Hence it was concluded that the muscle vasodilatation was simply a functional, or active, hyperaemia (see Chapter 7). By way of explanation for the earlier results, it is possible that stimulation in the cortex indirectly evoked the pattern of the alerting response, either by current spread to

pain afferents in the meninges, or from widespread discharges reaching the hypothalamus.

If we reject the idea that the alerting response can be elicited from the motor cortex, this does not mean that the pattern of the alerting response cannot precede exercise. Intuitively, it seems very unlikely that all exercise, even walking across a room or walking with the dog, is preceded by an alerting response. However, the alerting response could be evoked by other inputs to the defence areas if the exercise were anticipated and had an emotional component. Further, rejection of the motor cortex as an input to the defence areas certainly does not imply that other cortical areas have no influence over the defence areas, as is discussed below.

Evidence from chemical stimulation
The drawback of using electrical stimulation as a means of investigating the neural organization of any pattern of response is that the technique inevitably activates fibres of passage as well as cell bodies. This can be avoided by microapplication of excitatory amino acids that activate only cell bodies and dendrites. However, microapplication holds the disadvantage that the pattern of response observed may depend upon the spatial arrangement, density and cytoarchitecture of the neurones, and thereby on whether a sufficiently large pool of functionally homogeneous neurones can be stimulated together. With these provisos, recent studies in which amino acids have been employed have so far demonstrated that, in the Saffan-anaesthetized rat, the tachycardia and regional vascular components of the alerting response can be evoked by microinjection of D-L-homocysteic acid (DLH) into the basolateral nucleus of the amygdala [14] (Fig. 6). Arterial pressure tended to fall, but this could be explained by the rather larger muscle vasodilatation in comparison with the renal vasoconstriction. By contrast, chemical stimulation in the more dorsal, central nucleus of the amygdala produced no cardiovascular response, even though electrical stimulation at this region was effective in producing the full response. These findings suggest that neurones which make the appropriate connections for producing the cardiovascular pattern of the alerting response are present in the basal nucleus, while the central nucleus may lie on the afferent pathway to the

amygdala from the stria, or on the amygdalofugal pathway to the hypothalamus.

A cardiovascular response pattern comparable with that evoked from the basal nucleus of the amygdala has also been evoked by microinjection of DLH in the rostral hypothalamus, just dorsal to the optic chiasma, in the region that was identified by electrical stimulation (Fig. 6). In the conscious rat, DLH application in this same region elicited alerting behaviour and brisk locomotion [15]. However, injection of DLH into the perifornical region of the hypothalamus of the rat, in the region that has been considered of particular importance in the generation of the defence response, evoked muscle vasodilatation, tachycardia and all the behavioural signs of alerting that an anaesthetized animal is capable of showing, i.e. pupillary dilatation and exophthalmus, but no renal vasoconstriction. This has led to the suggestion that the role of the perifornical region should be reconsidered. Doubt was compounded by the fact that, in the conscious rat, injection of DLH into the perifornical region was not able to evoke the full behavioural signs of aggressive or defensive behaviour, a finding which has been confirmed in conscious cats [16].

It may be that 'defence neurones' are widely scattered in the perifornical region, or that this region largely comprises fibres of passage. Unfortunately, there has so far been no investigation with excitatory amino acids as to whether the full pattern of the alerting response can be evoked from the lateral hypothalamus or the band dorsal to the optic tract, where synapses on the pathway from the amygdala were predicted from the effects of anaesthetics (see above). It would certainly seem unwise to discard the idea that the hypothalamus serves as an integrative region for the alerting/defence response, given the fact that in decerebrate animals show a fully co-ordinated behavioural and cardiovascular response to noxious stimulation only occurs if the line of decerebration spares the hypothalamus (see above). The characteristics of the alerting defence response are listed in Table 2.

Injection of DLH into the dorsal periaqueductal grey matter of the midbrain and pons (Fig. 6) in the anaesthetized rat readily evoked the full cardiovascular pattern of the alerting response, including renal vasoconstriction and a rise in arterial pressure, and, in the conscious

Table 2. Characteristics of the alerting defence response

- Increased cardiac output
- Vasoconstriction in kidney, gastrointestinal tract and skin
- Vasodilatation in muscle
- Increased arterial pressure
- Pupillary dilatation, piloerection, urination and defaecation
- Common to mammalian species
- Appropriate stimulus varies between species
- Appropriate stimulus varies between individuals in a single species
- Response is graded with stimulus strength
- Response may outlast the stimulus
- During response, baroreceptor reflex suppressed in graded manner
- Response can show habituation or sensitization
- Response can be conditioned

rat, evoked behavioural patterns ranging from mild alerting to flight [15]. Similarly, chemical stimulation of the homologous region in the anaesthetized rabbit has been reported to evoke the cardiovascular components of the alerting response, while such stimulation in the conscious cat evoked threatening behaviour. Thus there is no doubt that this region contains neurones which can trigger the full behavioural and cardiovascular patterns of response. The effects of chemical stimulation in the more-lateral tegmental region of the pons were as equivocal as the responses evoked from the perifornical region of the hypothalamus. The dorsal medullary strip that was identified as part of the defence area has not been investigated using chemical stimulation.

If the effects of electrical and chemical stimulation are considered together, then it seems that the ideas put forward by Abrahams and co-workers in the 1960s are still acceptable; the defence regions from the preoptic region through the hypothalamus to the dorsal periaqueductal grey matter of the midbrain, and extending to the dorsal medulla, behave as an entity that can be activated by afferent inputs from the amygdala and periphery. This might be facilitated by reciprocal connections between the regions, for example, the hypothalamus and periaqueductal grey. On the other hand, it appears that the regions can also act independently. Therefore the full pattern of response can still be evoked from the hypothalamus after extensive lesions involving much of the dorsal midbrain, while animals in which the hypothalamus has been removed — by sectioning rostral to the periaqueductal grey — can show patterned defensive behaviour in response to strong noxious stimulation.

▶ The cardiovascular pattern of the alerting response, which is mediated by patterned changes in parasympathetic and sympathetic activity, is integrated in localized regions of the forebrain and brainstem, from the amygdala through the hypothalamus to the dorsal midbrain and medulla. All of these regions funnel into an efferent pathway which synapses onto neurones in the rostral ventrolateral medulla (RVLM).
▶ Experiments involving DLH, which stimulates cell bodies but not nerve fibres, indicate that the cell bodies of the neurones that mediate the alerting response are in the basal nucleus of the amygdala, possibly in the rostral hypothalamus, but certainly in the periaqueductal grey matter of the midbrain and medulla. The output from these regions can be modulated by inputs from frontal cortex and can modulate reflex pathways at the medullary level.

The ventral medulla

The activity from the defence areas apparently funnels through the single ventral medullary pathway, which has itself been the subject of recent investigation. Using electrical stimulation in the Althesin-anaesthetized cat, the full cardiovascular pattern of the alerting response could be evoked from a longitudinal strip running caudally through the midbrain and as far as a region just caudal to the trapezoid bodies (Fig. 7). At sites more caudal than this, electrical stimulation seemed to evoke individual components but not the whole pattern of the response. The region where the response seemed to fractionate corresponded closely with what had been called the 'glycine-sensitive area', since

bilateral application of glycine to this region produced respiratory apnoea and a dramatic fall in arterial pressure [17] (see Chapter 1). Since glycine depresses the activity of neuronal cell bodies, this implied that there are neurones in the glycine-sensitive area that play an important tonic excitatory role in setting the normal level of arterial pressure. However, Hilton and co-workers [18] also found that bilateral application of glycine, or application of glycine to one side and electrolytic lesion of the other, abolished the cardiovascular components of the alerting response evoked from the amygdala, hypothalamus or midbrain (Fig. 7), indicating that the ventral defence pathway synapses in these regions on to the neurones with tonic excitatory drive.

Since then, electrophysiological and neuronal tracing studies on this region, which is anatomically defined as the nucleus paragigantocellularis lateralis, but is now widely known as the RVLM (rostral ventrolateral medulla), have demonstrated that these neurones receive direct projections from the defence areas (Fig. 8) and also from many other regions of the brain, including the parabrachial nucleus, ventral periaqueductal grey matter and nucleus tractus solitarius (see Chapter 1, Fig. 4) and that they project to the intermediolateral cell column to the region of the sympathetic preganglionic neurones (see Chapter 1).

Furthermore, microinjection of excitatory amino acids into this region can selectively produce vasoconstriction in mesenteric or renal circulation, vasoconstriction or vasodilatation in muscle, tachycardia or bradycardia and other autonomically mediated responses, depending on exactly where the injection is made. The obvious conclusion is that these neurones are already functionally dedicated and represent a major pathway to the sympathetic preganglionic neurones that is used to generate different patterns of autonomic response; the alerting pattern is just one of these patterns (see Chapter 1).

It has been proposed that the neurones of the RVLM have their own intrinsic activity but that this activity is also constantly moderated by afferent inputs. In as much as the defence areas have activity in the waking state, which is raised in response to alerting or noxious stimuli, the defence areas may provide one of the excitatory inputs that not only produces a characteristic pattern of cardiovascular response,

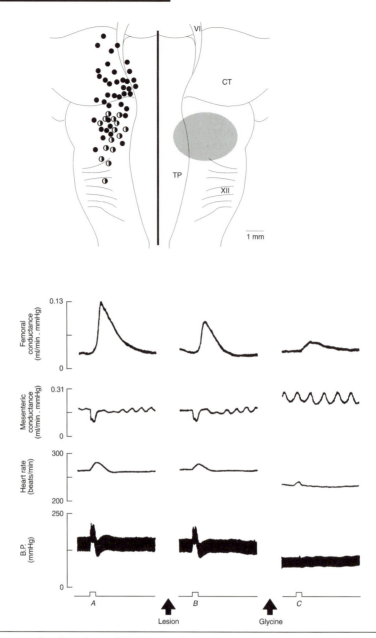

Fig. 7. A diagrammatic plan view of the ventral medulla of the cat (top) and the effects of an electrolytic lesion and glycine application to the ventral medullary surface on the alerting response evoked from the amygdala (bottom)

In the top diagram, filled circles indicate sites at which electrical stimulation evoked the full pattern of the alerting response; half-filled circles indicate sites at which electrical stimulation evoked responses similar to, but not identical with, the alerting response. The shaded area indicates the area to which glycine was applied. Abbreviations used: TP, pyramidal tract; CT, trapezoid body; VI and XII, abducens and hypoglossal nerves respectively. In the bottom diagram, traces show effects on resting levels of femoral (muscle) and mesenteric vascular conductance, heart rate and arterial blood pressure, and on changes evoked by stimulation in the amygdala of a ventral medullary lesion in the efferent pathway from the defence areas (middle) and of subsequent application of glycine to the contralateral glycine-sensitive area (right). Bars beneath traces indicate periods of stimulation. Modified and reproduced with permission from [17].

but contributes to the prevailing level of arterial pressure. However, it is also clear that the neurones of the RVLM are not the only excitatory pathway to the sympathetic preganglionic neurones. For example, bilateral application of glycine to the RVLM rapidly abolished the cardiovascular components of the alerting response evoked by peripheral chemoreceptor or radial nerve stimulation; but generalized vasoconstriction could be evoked by both stimuli until the arterial pressure became so low that the sympathetic preganglionic neurones were probably too far below their thresholds to be activated.

It should also be remembered that the role of the RVLM is not restricted to autonomic function. The surface of the ventral medulla has also been proposed as the site of central chemosensitivity to carbon dioxide. This has been questioned by some. However, it is clear that respiration is severely depressed or abolished by bilateral application of glycine to the RVLM, and by bilateral cooling or electrolytic lesion of this same region, and that this respira-

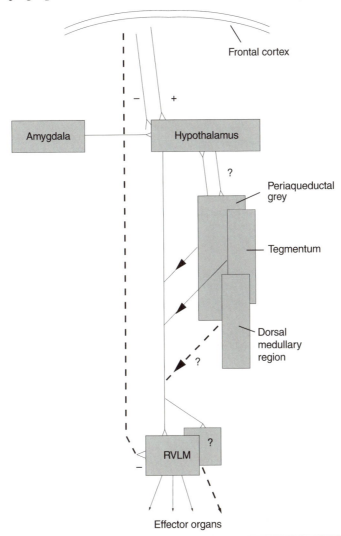

Fig. 8. **Schematic diagram showing the brain regions that are thought to be involved in the integration or modification of the alerting response**
+ *and* − *indicate excitatory and inhibitory influences, respectively. Dashed lines indicate proposed pathways. For further details, see text.*

tory depression is accompanied by loss of responsiveness to carbon dioxide. In fact, this region has been called Area S, or Intermediate Area, by those investigating central chemosensitivity. It obviously provides a major tonic excitatory drive to respiration and has been proposed as the site of relay from more caudal and rostral chemosensitive areas: Areas M and L, respectively [18].

Thus it seems likely that the RVLM is an important site of integration of cardiovascular and respiratory regulation. It is, therefore, particularly interesting that in the cat, inhalation of carbon dioxide not only caused the expected increased respiration, but reduced the muscle vasodilatation and enhanced the splanchnic vasoconstriction of the alerting response evoked by stimulation in the amygdala. Similar effects upon these cardiovascular changes were induced by superfusion of the ventral medulla with cerebrospinal fluid of low pH, while opposite effects were induced by superfusion with high pH. It may be that these effects are exerted by the modulatory influence of changes in pH upon synaptic transmission within the RVLM onto neurones that mediate the alerting response, rather than by effects on specific chemoreceptors for carbon dioxide, or hydrogen [19].

> ▶ The activity of the RVLM neurones, on to which the pathway for the alerting response synapse, provides a major tonic excitatory drive to sympathetic preganglionic neurones. Therefore, changes in the level of alertness, and thereby in the output from the defence areas to those medullary neurones, may play an important role in setting the level of arterial pressure.
> ▶ The region of the RVLM also contains neurones that are of major importance in the control of respiration. It seems probable that this ventral medullary region is an important site for integration of cardiovascular and respiratory function.

Habituation and sensitization of the response

The discussion so far may have given the impression that the cardiovascular pattern of the alerting response is stereotyped and consistent in response to a given stimulus. This may be true when the response is evoked by electrical or chemical stimulation in the brain. However, when evoked by more natural stimuli, in the conscious animal, the response pattern may show habituation or sensitization upon repetition of the stimulus [21]: habituation means that the response gradually becomes smaller, while sensitization means that it becomes larger. Of the two, habituation is the more common [21].

Habituation of the alerting response has been observed, for example, in the baboon when confronted by a snake, in the cat when confronted by a dog (Fig. 9), and in man when subjected to the cold pressor test (Fig. 10) or to auditory stimuli. Sensitization seems more likely to occur when the individual is already aroused or anxious, leading to the idea that this process is favoured when ongoing activity in the defence areas is high. It has been proposed that during repeated exposure to a given stimulus, the two processes of habituation and sensitization are activated in parallel within the central nervous system and that it is their interaction which determines the magnitude of the response observed. The outcome of this interaction is apparently dependent on the intensity and specificity of the stimulus, the frequency of repetition, as well as on the level of arousal of the individual [21].

Whether habituation or sensitization occurs in a given individual, there is not necessarily any correlation between the rate of change of the behavioural response and the cardiovascular response. Thus the magnitude of the behavioural response does not give a reliable indication of the cardiovascular response; it may persist when the cardiovascular response has been completely extinguished. In addition, the individual components of the cardiovascular response may change at different rates. Generally speaking, the muscle vasodilatation seems to be the component of the response that is most susceptible to habituation, and it may disappear completely at a time when the tachycardia, rise in arterial pressure, and renal and splanchnic vasoconstriction are almost as great as those seen in response to the first stimulus. On the other hand, experiments on dogs, baboons and human subjects suggest that in some individuals the renal vasoconstriction and other pressor components of the response habituate very readily as well [21].

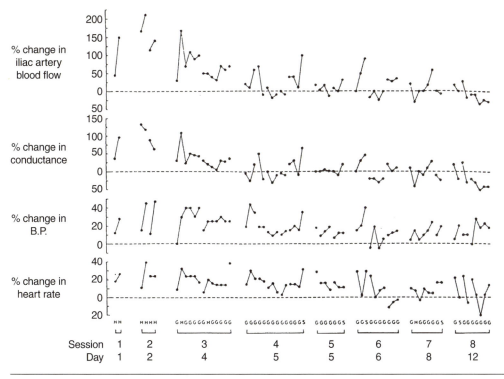

Fig. 9. **Habituation of the cardiovascular components of the alerting response evoked in a cat confronted by a dog**

*Each point corresponds to one bout of rage during confrontation. Abbreviations used: H, hissing; G, growling; S, striking with the front paw. Reproduced with permission from Martin, J., Sutherland, C.J. and Zbrozyna, A.W. (1976) Pfluegers Arch. **365** 37–47.*

▶ The alerting response can be habituated or sensitized on repetition of the stimulus. Individual components of the response may habituate or sensitize at different rates. The muscle vasodilatation seems the most vulnerable to both processes.

Hypertension

It has been proposed that those individuals who most readily develop renal vasoconstriction in response to aversive stimuli, and who show little or no habituation of it, are most likely to develop essential hypertension [4,21,22]. This is consistent with a large body of evidence suggesting that the defence response plays an important role in the genesis of essential hypertension. For example, the following observations have been made:

— hypertensive patients show a marked tendency towards nervous tension, anxiety, or so-called 'type A behaviour', and it has been found that conditioning, or yoga, can lower blood pressure in some hypertensives;

— labile hypertensives have a higher 'resting' level of muscle blood flow and muscle vascular conductance than normotensive subjects, which would be consistent with a high level of ongoing activity in the defence areas of the hypertensives (Fig. 10);

— labile hypertensives and established hypertensives show larger increases in muscle blood flow and muscle vascular conductance in response to stressful stimuli (Fig. 10), and the increases in arterial pressure evoked by mental stress are greater in labile hypertensives, and even in the normotensive, adolescent children of hypertensive subjects, than they are in normotensives with no family history of hypertension;

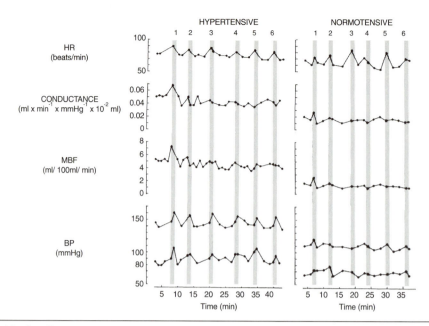

Fig. 10. Cardiovascular responses evoked in a hypertensive subject (left) and in a normotensive subject (right) on repeated immersion of one foot in cold water

Abbreviations used: BP, mean arterial pressure; MBF, forearm muscle blood flow; conductance, muscle vascular conductance calculated as MBF/BP; HR, heart rate.

*Reproduced with permission from Zbrozyna, A.W. and Krebbel, F. (1985). Eur. J. ppl. Physiol. **54**, 136–44.*

— the renal vasoconstrictor response to mental stress is more pronounced and longer lasting in established hypertensives than in normotensive subjects;

— while the muscle vasodilatation evoked by the cold pressor test showed some habituation in both labile hypertensives and normotensives, the increases in blood pressure, particularly the increases in diastolic pressure, remained of similar magnitude on repetition of the stimulus in the labile hypertensives, but gradually decreased in the normotensives, as would be consistent with lack of habituation of the renal vasoconstriction in the labile hypertensives (Fig 10).

Thus it seems that an individual who persistently shows pronounced alerting responses to the many unexpected and unpleasant stimuli of everyday life, and little habituation of the vasoconstrictor components, may be caught in a vicious circle. It is well-established that the increase in tension of blood vessel walls that results from increase of arterial pressure causes hypertrophy of the vascular smooth muscle

and, consequently, a reduction in vessel internal diameter, so providing a physical reason for increased vascular resistance and arterial pressure [22].

▶ There is evidence that the alerting response plays a role in the genesis of essential hypertension.

Central processing

The fact that the alerting response can show sensitization or habituation raises the possibility that there are regions of the brain that can increase or decrease the response by influencing the 'interpretation of the incoming sensory information', by altering the level of activity in the defence areas, or by modifying the outgoing pathway to the effectors. The fact that sensitization and habituation may have differential effects on individual components of the alerting response suggests that at least one of the sites of modification must be at a level within the central nervous system where there is separate representation of those individual components [21]. There has been relatively little experimental investigation of these possibilities. However, there is evidence from experiments on cats anaesthetized with Althesin that electrical stimulation within restricted regions of the frontal cortex produced no measurable cardiovascular responses when applied alone, but caused a significant reduction of the cardiovascular components of an alerting response evoked by simultaneous stimulation of the amygdala, the muscle vasodilatation being affected most [23]. Since stimulation at these same cortical sites had no effect on the alerting response evoked by stimulation in the hypothalamus, it seems likely that the modulating influence is exerted at synapses in the efferent pathway from the amygdala to the hypothalamus (Fig. 8). On the other hand, stimulation at other sites within a different region of the frontal cortex substantially facilitated the amygdaloid response, with no effect on the hypothalamic response, suggesting that the cortex can also facilitate synaptic transmission in the amygdalo-hypothalamic pathway (Fig. 8).

In contrast, experiments on rats anaesthetized with Saffan showed that electrical or chemical stimulation with DLH within a restricted region of the frontal cortex had no cardiovascular effect when applied alone, but reduced or abolished both the muscle vasodilator and renal vasoconstrictor components of the alerting response evoked from both the amygdala and the hypothalamus [24]. Since stimulation at the effective sites inhibited the alerting response evoked from the hypothalamus, as well as from the amygdala, the site of inhibition must be at synapses in the efferent pathway from these areas. The only site of synapses in the pathway from the defence areas that has been identified is in the RVLM (see Fig. 6), where the fibres synapse onto neurons that descend to produce the individual components of the response; this must, therefore, be a favoured site. The fact that stimulation in the frontal cortex alone had no detectable effect on cardiovascular variables suggests that the inhibitory influence is presynaptic. Interestingly, it has been shown in the rat that lesions of the frontal cortex can prevent habituation of the tachycardia evoked by noxious stimuli, while electrical stimulation in this region accelerated habituation of this response.

> ▶ The output from the defence areas of the brainstem can be modulated by inputs from the frontal cortex, and can modulate cardiovascular reflex pathways at the medullary level, probably at the RVLM. Such modulation may underlie habituation and sensitization.

Functional importance of the alerting response

It has been argued that the cardiovascular pattern of the alerting response provides a split-second advantage in a life-threatening situation by ensuring an increased nutritional supply to muscle even before exercise, defensive or aggressive behaviour begins. This is open to discussion, since functional or active hyperaemia begins immediately the muscle contracts. In any case, in the initial period of muscle contraction, muscle metabolism is not limited by oxygen supply (see Chapter 7). It may be that vasodilatation of the arteriolar vessels of muscle is more important in allowing the venous vessels to fill, so that as soon as the muscles contract, the skeletal muscle pump provides an immediate increase in venous return to the heart and a consequent increase in cardiac output according to Starling's Law.

On the other hand, it can also be argued that this response pattern is a potential threat to life. For example, the acute rise in arterial pressure is hazardous to an individual who is stroke-prone or has impaired coronary circulation, while repetition of the response in individuals who show little habituation may lead to the development of hypertension.

'Playing dead' or 'vasovagal syncope'

Although the pattern of the alerting response may be the most common and well-known response to novel, noxious or emotional stimuli, it is clear that under some conditions a very different pattern of response occurs. Playing dead seems to be particularly common in some species, for example, in the opossum (from which we get the expression 'playing possum'), in the rabbit and in deer fawn. This behavioural response is accompanied by bradycardia and a decrease in respiration. The term vasovagal syncope is used to describe sudden fainting, associated with a fall in arterial pressure, which results from bradycardia and vasodilatation. It is known to occur in human subjects who experience what is, to them, an extremely stressful situation from which there is no escape; for example, the sight of blood, news of the death of a close relative or the thought of a danger that must be faced can serve as triggers. It is not clear whether, from the point of view of the underlying physiological mechanisms, playing dead and the vasovagal syncope are the same response. However, it has been said that both occur in situations when 'looking dead is preferable to being dead'. The discussion that follows is mainly concerned with the vasovagal syncope in human subjects, because this has received more attention.

True emotional fainting is difficult to evoke under laboratory conditions. For some of the classical experiments in the field (Fig. 11), the investigators selected medical students who knew that they were likely to faint at the sight of blood. On finding that fainting did not occur in the laboratory when blood was removed from the subject by venepuncture, the investigators insisted that they would make the subject drink the blood — a faint ensued! Such experiments clearly demonstrated that before the faint there was an increase in arterial pressure, tachycardia and vasodilatation in forearm muscles, as would be expected during the alerting response. Then, suddenly, as if at the flick of a switch, there was pronounced bradycardia, further vasodilatation in the forearm and a fall in arterial pressure culminating in the faint [25]. It has been established that the bradycardia is mainly due to activation of the cardiac vagal fibres, while the vasodilatation in muscle has been attributed to inhibition of sympathetic noradrenergic fibre activity and to the actions of circulating adrenaline (Fig. 12). It has been claimed that the muscle vasodilatation is also mediated by increased sympathetic cholinergic activity, but acceptance of this idea is open to similar criticisms as discussed above in connection with the proposed involvement of sympathetic cholinergic fibres in the alerting response.

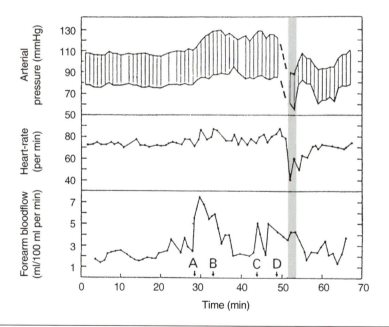

Fig. 11. **Cardiovascular changes in a male student during vasovagal syncope**
The student showed forearm vasodilatation and tachycardia as part of the alerting response while watching the preparation for venepuncture (A) and venepuncture of a colleague (B); however, he did not faint as he had on an earlier occasion. Insertion of a needle into his own arm (C) again produced forearm vasodilatation, but no faint. When he was asked to drink some of the blood taken from his colleague (D), he yawned and then fainted (stippled area). No heart beat was detectable for 11 s and then heart rate was 37 beats/min. Forearm blood flow remained well above the resting level despite the profound fall in arterial pressure, showing that vasodilatation had occurred. Consciousness was regained after 2 min. Reproduced with permission from [25].

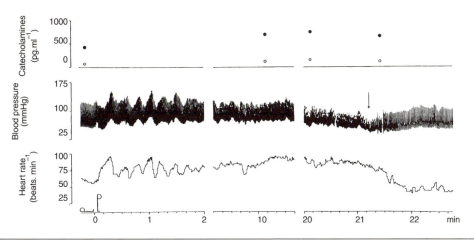

Fig. 12. Cardiovascular and plasma catecholamine changes recorded from a 40-year-old woman during vasovagal syncope induced by prolonged standing

Upon standing up (at time 0) there was an increase in heart rate and arterial pressure (recorded non-invasively). By 11 min, when heart rate had reached an even higher level, there was an increase in both plasma noradrenaline (○) and adrenaline (●) levels. Thereafter, plasma noradrenaline did not rise further, despite the gradual fall in arterial pressure and heart rate, while the rise in plasma adrenaline was maintained. At 21 min of standing, both heart rate and arterial pressure declined more rapidly until fainting occurred (arrow). At this time plasma adrenaline was still above the baseline level. After transition to the supine position at 21.2 min, arterial pressure rose again towards the original control level (before time 0). Reproduced with permission from Van Lieshout, J.J. (1989) Cardiovascular reflexes in orthostatic disorders. PhD Thesis, University of Amsterdam.

From a haemodynamic point of view, the vasovagal syncope evoked by strong emotion seems to be identical with the vasovagal syncope evoked by other stimuli that are far easier to use in the laboratory, for example, prolonged standing, particularly in a hot environment, passive head-up tilt or lower body negative pressure. An apparently similar response can also occur after heavy exercise, if the individual stops exercising suddenly and attempts to stand upright. Bradycardia, peripheral vasodilatation and syncope have also been reported when a large haemorrhage occurs over a short period of time. Further, a persistent slow heart rate together with a low arterial pressure is sometimes noted in otherwise healthy subjects who have suffered blood loss as a result of an accident (see Chapter 8), even though under these conditions one might expect a baroreceptor-mediated tachycardia as a reflex response to the hypotension. Whatever the provoking stimulus, it seems that vasovagal syncope is preceded by profuse sweating, nausea, yawning and pupillary dilatation, which supports the idea that we are dealing with the same response.

It is known from experiments on anaesthetized animals that electrical stimulation in a localized region of the hypothalamus, lateral to the 'defence area', evokes a pattern of bradycardia and peripheral vasodilatation which leads to a fall in arterial pressure. It is possible that this region contains the neurones that are involved in integrating the pattern of the vasovagal syncope, or that it contains the efferent pathway from an integrating region, as described above for the defence areas. The sudden switch from the alerting response to vasovagal syncope in acute emotional stress might be explained if the defence areas 'trigger' the area concerned with the vasovagal syncope. Alternatively, it may be that the area concerned with vasovagal syncope is itself activated by emotional inputs, but has a higher threshold to them than the defence areas. Neither of these ideas has been tested experimentally.

However, there is experimental evidence that the vasovagal syncope can be elicited by a discrete group of cardiac afferent fibres whose endings are in the walls of the ventricles [26]. These unmyelinated afferent fibres seem to be particularly sensitive to ventricular wall deformation and the inotropic state of cardiac muscle and are thought to be activated when the ventricles contract forcefully around a relatively small ventricular volume. Further, when cardiac afferent fibres are stimulated experimentally with stimulus parameters that are sufficiently strong to stimulate the unmyelinated afferent fibres (in addition to the myelinated fibres), then reflex bradycardia mediated by vagal efferent fibres, vasodilatation that is pronounced in skeletal muscle and a fall in arterial pressure occur. It may be noted that all of the conditions mentioned above as triggers for the vasovagal syncope (prolonged standing, head-up tilt, lower body negative pressure, a rapid large haemorrhage and cessation of heavy exercise) are likely to involve powerful contraction of the ventricular muscle, induced by sympathetic stimulation at a time when ventricular volume is relatively small because of venous pooling, loss of vascular volume or peripheral vasodilatation. Thus, they all have the potential to activate the ventricular afferents and elicit the vasovagal syncope as a reflex response. It may even be that emotional stress not only induces vasovagal syncope by the central mechanisms considered above, but that powerful contraction of the ventricular muscle and muscle vasodilatation elicited as part of the alerting response to emotional stress can, in extreme circumstances, result in the ventricles contracting around a small volume. In other words, it may be impossible to separate the central and reflex mechanisms.

▶ The vasovagal syncope may occur in extreme emotional stress, but also in conditions in which there is substantial venous pooling in dependent regions or rapid, major loss of blood. This response comprises a profound fall in arterial pressure caused by bradycardia and vasodilatation that is pronounced in skeletal muscle. These components are mediated by an increase in cardiac vagal activity and a decrease in sympathetic vasoconstrictor nerve activity.
▶ The response may be triggered by emotional inputs to an integrating area in the forebrain, but also by cardiac ventricular afferents that are stimulated when the ventricle contracts strongly around a small volume.

Functionally, the vasovagal syncope may be a disadvantage after a severe haemorrhage in that it antagonizes the baroreceptor reflex and accentuates the fall in arterial pressure. However, it may serve a useful function in protecting the heart by rapidly reducing myocardial oxygen demand when cardiac work is excessive. Moreover, fainting itself, if it puts the body ina supine position, certainly allows for a better filling of the heart and restoration of arterial pressure.

References

1. Hilton, S.M. (1982) The defence arousal system and its relevance for circulatory and respiratory control. J. Exp. Biol. 100, 159–174
2. Uvnas, B. (1970) Cholinergic muscle vasodilatation. In Cardiovascular regulation in health and disease. (Bartorelli, C. and Zanchetti, A., eds.), pp. 7–16, Cardiovascular Research Institute, Milan
3. Caraffa-Braga, E., Granata, L. and Pinotti, O. (1973) Changes in blood flow distribution during acute emotional stress in dogs. Pfluegers Arch. 339, 203–316
4. Brod, J., Fencl, V., Hejl, Z. and Jirka, J. (1959) Circulatory changes underlying blood pressure elevation during acute emotional stress (mental arithmetic) in normotensive and hypertensive subjects. Clin. Sci. 18, 269–279
5. Yardley, C.P. and Hilton, S.M. (1987) Vasodilatation in hind limb skeletal muscle evoked as part of the defence reaction in the rat. J. Auton. Nerv. Syst. 19, 127–136
6. Shimada, S.G. and Stitt, J.T. (1984) Analysis of the purinergic component of active muscle vasodilatation of the defence response. Brit. J. Pharmacol. 83, 577–589
7. Barcroft, H., Brod, J., Hejl, Z., Hirsjarvi, E.A. and Kitchin, A.H. (1960) The mechanism of the vasodilatation in the forearm muscles during stress (mental arithmetic). Clin. Sci. 19, 577–586
8. Timms, R.J. (1981) A study of the amygdaloid defence reaction showing the value of Althesin in studies of the function of the forebrain in cats. Pfluegers Arch. 391, 49–56
9. Marshall, J.M. (1987) Contribution to overall cardiovascular control made by the chemoreceptor-induced defence response. In The Neurobiology of the Cardiorespiratory System (Taylor, E.W., ed.), pp. 222–240, Manchester University Press, Manchester
10. Marshall J.M. and Metcalfe, J.D. (1990) Effects of systemic hypoxia on the distribution of cardiac output in the rat. J. Physiol. 426, 335–353
11. Kylstra, P.H. and Lisander, B. (1970) Differential interaction between the hypothalamic defence area and baroreceptor reflexes. Acta Physiol. Scand. 78, 386–392
12. Coote, J.H., Hilton, S.M. and Perez-Gonzalez, J.F. (1979) Inhibition of the baroreceptor reflex on stimulation in the brain stem defence centre. J. Physiol. 288, 549–560
13. Hilton, S.M., Spyer, K.M. and Timms, R.J. (1979) The origin of the hindlimb vasodilatation evoked by stimulation of the motor cortex in the cat. J. Physiol. 287, 545–557
14. Maskati, H.A.A. and Zbrozyna, A.W. (1989) Cardiovascular and motor components of the defence reaction elicited in rats by electrical and chemical stimulation in amygdala. J. Auton. Nerv. Syst. 28, 127–132

15. Hilton, S.M. and Redfern, W. (1986) A search for brain stem cell groups integrating the defence reaction in the rat. J. Physiol. **378**, 213–228

16. Jordan, D. (1990) Autonomic changes in affective behaviour. In Central regulation of autonomic function (Loewy, A.D. and Spyer, K.M.), pp. 349–366, Oxford University Press, Oxford

17. Guertzenstein, P.G. and Silver, A. (1974) Fall in blood pressure produced from discrete regions of the ventral surface of the medulla by glycine and lesions. J. Physiol. **242**, 489–503

18. Hilton, S.M., Marshall, J.M. and Timms, R.J. (1983) Ventral medullary relay neurones in the pathway from the defence areas of the cat and their effect on blood pressure. J. Physiol. **345**, 149–166

19. Marshall J.M. (1986) The role of the glycine-sensitive area of the ventral medulla in cardiovascular responses to carotid chemoreceptor and peripheral nerve stimulation. Pfluegers Arch. **406**, 226–231

20. Marshall J.M. (1986) Modulation of the centrally-evoked visceral alerting response by changes in CSF pH at the ventral surface of the medulla oblongata and by systemic hypercapnia. Pfluegers Arch. **407**, 46–54

21. Zbrozyna, A.W. Habituation of cardiovascular responses. In Neurobiology of the Cardiorespiratory System. (Taylor, E.W. ed.), pp. 241–260, Manchester University Press, Manchester

22. Folkow, B. (1978) Cardiovascular structural adaptation; its role in the initiation and maintenance of primary hypertension. Clin. Sci. Mol. Med. **55**, 3s–22s

23. Timms, R.J. (1977) Cortical inhibition and facilitation of the defence reaction. J. Physiol. **266**, 98–99

24. Maskati, H.A.A. and Zbrozyna, A.W. (1989) Stimulation in prefrontal cortex area inhibits cardiovascular and motor components of the defence reaction in rats. J. Auton. Nerv. Syst. **28**, 117–126

25. Greenfield, A.D.M. (1951) An emotional faint. Lancet **i**, 1302–1303

26. Thoren, P. (1979) Role of cardiac vagal C-fibres in cardiovascular control. Rev. Physiol. Biochem. Pharmacol. **86**, 1–94

Cardiovascular changes associated with sleep

Janice M. Marshall
Department of Physiology, The Medical School, Birmingham B15 2TT, U.K.

Introduction

Sleep is generally divided into several stages, on the basis of the activity recorded in the electroencephalogram (EEG). The waking state is characterized by the low-voltage, fast electrical activity of the cerebral cortex and subcortical structures, which is desynchronized. The first phase of drowsiness and sleep is associated with some loss of tone in postural muscles and with the appearance of groups of waves with a frequency of 8–12 Hz (spindles) on a background of high-voltage, slow waves in the EEG. This phase can be divided into stages 1–4 in man, but is generally known as light, synchronized or slow-wave sleep. It is replaced at intervals by the appearance of low-voltage, high-frequency activity in the EEG, which is indistinguishable from that occurring in the awake state, yet the individual is more difficult to arouse. There is also an almost complete loss of tone in postural muscles, apart from brief episodes when there are rapid eye movements, associated with twitches of the head, trunk and limbs and dreaming. This type of sleep is variously known as deep, desynchronized, paradoxical, or rapid eye movement (REM) sleep, and is further divided into tonic and phasic periods which coincide with muscle atonia and with muscle and ocular movements, respectively.

Synchronized and desynchronized sleep alternate in an irregular way, synchronized sleep normally being the first step of the cycle. The length of each cycle varies considerably between species; from the beginning of synchronized sleep to the end of desynchronized sleep is about 10 min in the rat, 25 min in the cat and 90 min in man. Studies on man have shown that the length of each period of desynchronized sleep increases as the night progresses, so that this type of sleep dominates in the early morning.

Arterial pressure

It has been known since the end of the last century that arterial pressure falls during sleep. However, the first detailed analyses of the changes in arterial pressure that occur during the various stages of sleep were carried out in the 1960s by Zanchetti and colleagues [1]. In their very thorough and extensive work on instrumented cats, they showed that during synchronized sleep arterial pressure fell by a few millimetres of Hg from that recorded during quiet wakefulness and there was a decrease in arterial pressure variability (Fig. 1). During the tonic phase of desynchronized sleep, there was a further, more marked fall in arterial pressure, by about 15%, from the quiet wakefulness value, i.e. from a mean value of 98 mmHg to 82 mmHg. However, during the phasic periods of desynchronized sleep, there were sharp increases in arterial pressure, coinciding with the bursts of eye movement and muscle twitches. In fact, during these phasic episodes, arterial pressure rose towards or even above the level recorded during quiet wakefulness, while during the tonic periods, arterial pressure reached the lowest levels of the circadian cycle (Fig. 1). Thus arterial pressure was far more variable during desynchronized sleep: the pressure range being about three times greater than during synchronized sleep.

Similar changes in arterial pressure have been recorded in a range of species, including the opossum, rabbit, dog and rhesus monkey [2]. For man also there is general agreement that arterial pressure falls during synchronized sleep. There have been reports that arterial pressure rises in man during desynchronized sleep. However, this conclusion seems to arise from attempts to calculate a mean level of arterial pressure at a time when arterial pressure is very variable. In fact, arterial pressure reaches its lowest levels during the tonic periods of desynchronized sleep, and rises towards the waking level during the phasic periods. However, the phasic periods occupy a greater part of the total time, at least in comparison with the cat, so that the falls in arterial pressure are less obvious and make a smaller contribution to a calculated mean. The rat also shows an

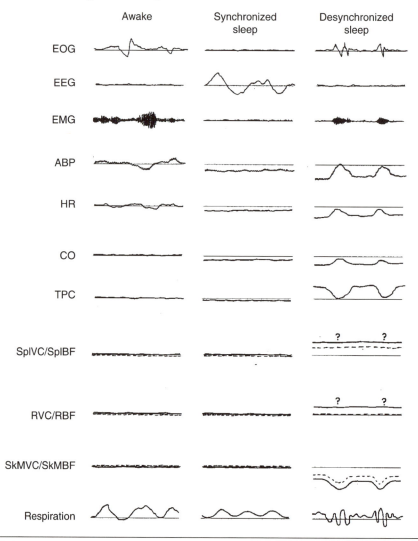

Fig. 1. **Schematic diagrams showing the characteristics of the awake state, synchronized sleep and the tonic and phasic components of desynchronized sleep**

Abbreviations used: EOG, electro-oculogram; EEG, electroencephalogram; EMG, electromyogram; ABP, arterial blood pressure; HR, heart rate; CO, cardiac output; TPC, total peripheral conductance; SplVC/SplBF, splanchnic vascular conductance and blood flow; RVC/RBF, renal vascular conductance and blood flow; SkMVC/SkMBF, skeletal muscle vascular conductance and blood flow. Vascular conductances and blood flows are shown by continuous and dotted lines, respectively. Respiration is respiratory air flow. The EOG and EMG activity during desynchronized sleep represent the phasic periods of desynchronized sleep. Question marks indicate that no recordings have been made of the changes that occur in splanchnic and renal vascular conductances and blood flows in phasic desynchronized sleep.

increase rather than a decrease in arterial pressure during desynchronized sleep. This may also be attributed to a greater time spent in the phasic periods of desynchronized sleep. Another possibility is that it simply reflects a difference in the balance of excitatory and inhibitory influences upon the cardiovascular system of the rat, as compared with some other species (see below).

Cardiac and peripheral vascular changes

Recordings on a large number of species have shown that heart rate falls during synchronized sleep and becomes very variable during desynchronized sleep (Fig. 1). Detailed studies on the cat have demonstrated that the changes in heart rate closely parallel the changes in arterial pressure, there being a small reduction in synchronized sleep, by a maximum of 8 beats per min, a further fall during the tonic periods of desynchronized sleep, by up to 18 beats per min, with a marked rise in heart rate coinciding with each phasic period [1]. Continuous recordings made from electromagnetic flow probes implanted on the ascending aorta of cats demonstrated that cardiac output fell during synchronized sleep and fell further during the tonic phases of desynchronized sleep. These changes in cardiac output were not accompanied by any consistent changes in stroke volume.

Calculations from measurements of arterial pressure and cardiac output indicated that, during synchronized sleep, total peripheral conductance changes little and may even fall slightly, demonstrating that the fall in arterial pressure during this type of sleep must be entirely due to the fall in cardiac output. On the other hand, during the tonic part of desynchronized sleep, calculated total peripheral conductance rose substantially, to the extent that this was largely responsible for the fall in arterial pressure (Fig. 1).

Clearly, an increase in total peripheral conductance (conductance = 1/resistance, see Glossary) implies a net vasodilatation in the peripheral vascular beds. However, this was not a generalized effect [1]. During synchronized sleep, electromagnetic blood flow recordings made from major arteries in the cat showed no consistent changes in splanchnic, renal or in hindlimb blood flow. Nevertheless, during the tonic periods of desynchronized sleep, there was a substantial increase in splanchnic and renal vascular conductance, indicating vasodilatation, whereas limb vascular conductance showed a pronounced decrease, indicating vasoconstriction. In the splanchnic circulation, the vasodilatation led to a substantial increase in blood flow, while in the kidney, blood flow remained more or less constant (Fig. 1). The decrease in hindlimb vascular conductance persisted when the paw was ligated, demonstrating that the vasoconstriction was in muscle rather than in skin. Indeed, studies in which cutaneous vascular responses have been assessed from changes in skin temperature, or paw volume, have suggested that the skin, like splanchnic circulation, shows little change during synchronized sleep and vasodilatation, with an increase in blood flow during the tonic periods of desynchronized sleep. Similar recordings made in the dog suggested that the regional vascular changes that occur in this species during synchronized and desynchronized sleep are comparable with those of the cat.

Again, the phasic periods of desynchronized sleep have to be considered separately, for the recordings on the cat showed that during these periods total peripheral conductance decreased, implying net vasoconstriction; this was largely due to further vasoconstriction in muscle. Interestingly, more-detailed analyses of muscle vasculature performed using an isotope dilution technique revealed that muscle vasoconstriction during the tonic periods of desynchronized sleep occurred predominantly in red, rather than white muscles [3]. Since red muscles are responsible for postural tone, this accords well with the loss of postural tone during tonic, desynchronized sleep. On the other hand, recent studies using the same technique have suggested that the blood flow to white muscles is increased during desynchronized sleep, raising the possibility that there is vasodilatation in white muscle. This may be explained as a functional or active hyperaemia, secondary to muscle contraction (see Chapter 7), as the muscular twitches that occur during the phasic periods of desynchronized sleep are, at least in part, due to contraction of white muscles.

It is not surprising that few studies have been performed on the regional vascular changes that occur in man during sleep, given that venous occlusion plethysmography, the method that has been readily available to assess peripheral blood flow, provides only discontinuous measurements and involves the inflation of vascular occluding cuffs, which is itself likely to disturb the pattern of sleep. However, there is evidence that cardiac output does not fall during synchronized sleep in man, indicating that the fall in arterial pressure reflects net peripheral vasodilatation. Moreover, plethysmography applied to the fingers showed little change during synchronized sleep, but suggested that cutaneous vasodilatation occurred during the tonic periods of desynchronized sleep, and cutaneous vasoconstriction during the phasic periods, similar to the observations made in the cat. Recent recordings [4], by plethysmography, of forearm and calf blood flows showed that there were large variations in blood flow and vascular conductance, in both regions that were independent of one another. These variations were much greater than the variations seen during quiet wakefulness and showed no obvious correlation with the stage of sleep. In other words, both increases and decreases in vascular conductance were seen in

forearm and in calf during both synchronized and desynchronized sleep; no attempt was made to analyse separately the phasic and tonic periods of desynchronized sleep.

The mediation of the efferent pattern of cardiovascular response

The fall in heart rate that occurs in synchronized sleep has been attributed predominantly to an increase in cardiac vagal activity, although there may also be a reduction in cardiac sympathetic activity (Fig. 2). Different research groups have ascribed the further fall in heart rate during the tonic periods of desynchronized sleep either to a further increase in vagal activity or to inhibition of sympathetic activity (Fig. 3). It seems likely that both occur, since the bradycardia cannot be abolished unless both the vagal and sympathetic influences on the heart are blocked. Further, it seems that the increases in heart rate that occur during the phasic periods of desynchronized sleep are due to reciprocal changes in vagal and sympathetic activity.

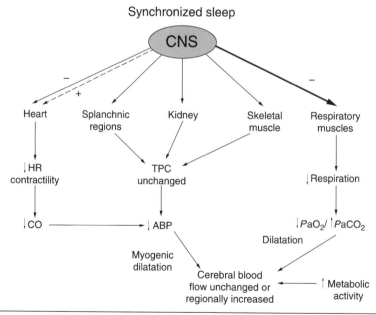

Fig. 2. **Schematic diagram indicating the respiratory and cardiovascular changes that occur during synchronized sleep**

Thin continuous and dotted lines from CNS (central nervous system) indicate sympathetic and parasympathetic fibres, respectively; thick continuous line indicates somatic motor fibres; + and − indicate increase and decrease in activity, respectively; arrows by variables indicate direction of change in the variable. See Fig. 1 for abbreviations used.

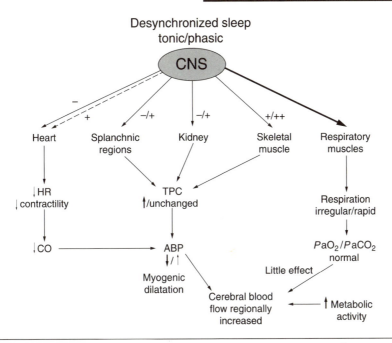

Fig. 3. **Schematic diagram indicating the respiratory and cardiovascular changes that occur during the tonic and phasic periods of desynchronized sleep**

Symbols and abbreviations as in Fig. 2. In each case, when the changes that occur in the tonic and phasic periods differ, the change in the tonic periods is given first and that in the phasic periods is given second, the thickness of the arrows indicating the magnitude of the change.

The rather fragmentary evidence available suggests that differential changes in the activity of the sympathetic nervous system are responsible for the peripheral vascular changes that occur during sleep [1,2] (Figs. 2 and 3). Thus total sympathectomy virtually abolished the increase in peripheral vascular conductance that occurred in the cat during tonic, desynchronized sleep. Recordings from the renal sympathetic nerves during natural sleep in cats demonstrated no change, or a slight decrease in activity in synchronized sleep, but a large decrease in activity in desynchronized sleep which was interrupted by bursts of activity that coincided with the phasic periods of desynchronized sleep. Further, sympathectomy of one hindlimb blocked the vasoconstriction that normally occurred in that limb during tonic desynchronized sleep, indicating that it was mediated by an increase in sympathetic noradrenergic activity.

The role of the sympathetic nervous system was investigated in a different way by Futuro-Neto and Coote [5,6]. They used unanaesthetized cats which had been decerebrated at the intercollicular level. Such preparations spontaneously go into a state that resembles desynchronized sleep, judging from the decreased extensor rigidity, rapid eye movements, and cardiovascular changes, and these are thought to be caused by the same central nervous structures that are responsible for desynchronized sleep in the intact animal. The carotid sinus nerves and aortic nerves were cut so as to accentuate the cardiovascular changes (see below) and under these conditions it was found that the desynchronized sleep-like periods were accompanied, during the tonic periods, by a decrease in cardiac sympathetic activity, a decrease in renal, splanchnic and lumbar sympathetic activity, and by an increase in the sympathetic activity to skeletal muscle, exactly as would be predicted from the vascular conductance changes recorded in the intact animal.

The changes that occurred during the phasic periods of desynchronized sleep have also been investigated. In the cat, the further muscle vasoconstriction was abolished by sympathectomy, indicating that it was mediated by an increase in sympathectomy activity. In addition, in the decerebrate cat, phasic increases in cardiac renal, splanchnic, lumbar and muscle sympathetic activity were observed during desynchronized-sleep-like periods.

> ▶ The transition from wakefulness to sleep is accompanied by a small fall in arterial pressure in synchronized sleep and by a further, larger fall in arterial pressure in the tonic phases of desynchronized sleep due to bradycardia, vasodilatation in splanchnic, cutaneous and renal vasculature, and vasoconstriction in skeletal muscle.
> ▶ During the phasic periods of desynchronized sleep, arterial pressure rises towards waking values, attributable to further vasoconstriction in muscle. These changes can all be attributed to patterned changes in sympathetic and cardiac vagal activity.

Respiratory changes

Although this chapter is mainly concerned with the cardiovascular changes that accompany sleep, it is important to give some consideration to the ways in which the pattern of respiration is changed, first, because the functioning of the cardiovascular and respiratory system is generally thought to be closely linked (see Chapter 2) and, secondly, because the respiratory changes have a bearing on the changes that occur in the cerebral circulation (see below).

Breathing rate has been recorded during sleep in many species, including rat, opossum, cat, dog, sheep, cow, horse, monkey and man [2,7]. There is general agreement that breathing rate decreases during synchronized sleep and that breathing becomes far more regular than during quiet wakefulness. However, expiratory pauses also occur, as do periodic fluctuations in the depth of breathing, and these are superimposed on the decreased rate. Measurements of tidal volume made in cat, dog and man showed a small mean increase in tidal volume during synchronized sleep but, overall, the decrease in rate resulted in a fall in minute ventilation. This in turn can be attributed, in part, to a reduction in metabolic activity, since oxygen consumption fell, while carbon dioxide production decreased. However, the fall in minute ventilation cannot be totally attributed to a fall in metabolic activity, as the partial pressure of arterial carbon dioxide ($PaCO_2$) rises in synchronized sleep by 5–6 mmHg, while PaO_2 can fall by up to 10 mmHg (Fig. 2).

The characteristic feature of breathing in desynchronized sleep is that it is irregular and rapid (Fig. 1). More-detailed analysis shows that there are periods of regular respiration and apnoea, but they are frequently broken by periods of hyperventilation. There is some evidence that the periods of hyperventilation are associated with periods of phasic sleep. Overall, minute ventilation increases towards that seen in the awake state, so that $PaCO_2$ and PaO_2 approach the awake values (Fig. 3).

> ▶ Breathing is depressed during synchronized sleep, but becomes rapid and irregular during desynchronized sleep.

Cerebral blood flow

In the awake state, brain vasculature is strongly influenced by changes in $PaCO_2$ and in perfusion pressure. Hypercapnia, or a fall in perfusion pressure, induces cerebral vasodilatation, but, whereas hypercapnia may actually increase brain blood flow, the myogenic dilator response to a fall in perfusion pressure tends to keep brain blood flow constant. Brain vasculature is also influenced by local changes in neuronal activity, an increase in activity leading to a local vasodilatation and increase in blood flow (see Chapter 7). Thus it might be expected that all of these influences would be important during sleep.

To some extent, this seems to be true, although the studies that have been carried out have been limited by the difficulties of recording cerebral blood flow continuously and regionally, and of obtaining reliable and regional measurements of cerebral metabolism. Notably, many of the techniques available only provide three or four single measurements in an individual animal, or only provide measurements in superficial regions of the brain.

One of the most detailed studies carried out on the cat by using the antipyrine autoradiographic technique [8] which allows regional blood flows to be measured, showed that synchronized sleep was accompanied by increases in blood flow in 10 of the 25 regions studied. These regions included the reticular formation, cochlear, cerebellar and vestibular nuclei, inferior and superior olives, hypothalamus, amygdala and association cortex, and the flow increases ranged from 26–68% (Fig. 4). However, there was no change in flow in the hippocampus, thalamus, caudate nucleus, lateral and medial geniculate, or in the visual, auditory, sensory and motor cortex. These differential effects may reflect increases in metabolic activity in the former group and no change, or a decrease in metabolism of the latter group. It is also possible that in the latter group blood flow was prevented from falling with the

fall in arterial pressure by myogenic dilatation caused by the fall in perfusion pressure and by vasodilatation induced by the rise in $PaCO_2$ (see Chapter 7) that occurs during synchronized sleep (see above).

The changes that occur during desynchronized sleep are far more dramatic. A range of studies on human subjects and on several animal species, involving several different techniques, have demonstrated that there are large increases in blood flow in the cerebral cortex as well as in other parts of the brain. Notably, in the study on the cat, blood flow increased during desynchronized sleep in all regions studied, ranging from 60% in the cerebellar white matter to 170% in the cochlear nuclei, the largest increases generally being in the brainstem structures (Fig. 4). Since there is no consistent change in $PaCO_2$ during desynchronized sleep (see above), and since a fall in arterial

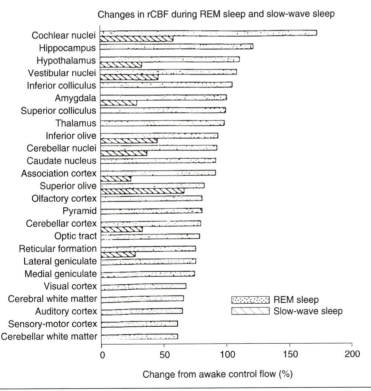

Fig. 4. The effect of synchronized (slow-wave) and desynchronized (REM) sleep on regional cerebral blood flow (rCBF) in cats expressed as a percentage change from the awake state

Reproduced with permission from Reivich, M. (1968) In Cerebral Vascular Diseases (Toole, J.F., Seikert, R.G. and Whisant, J.P., eds.), pp. 91–100, Grune and Stratton, New York

pressure would only be expected — by myogenic dilatation — to preserve a constant blood flow, it seems likely that these increases in cerebral blood flow reflect vasodilatation due to regional increases in metabolic activity. Evidence that cerebral metabolic activity is increased during desynchronized sleep is at the present time indirect, or circumstantial. However, there is plenty of evidence that neuronal activity is increased during the desynchronized sleep, for example, in the cortex, thalamus, hippocampus, hypothalamus and regionally within the brainstem, suggesting that associated increases in metabolic activity are waiting to be demonstrated. It is possible that activation of dilator nerve fibres contributes to the cerebral vasodilatation (see Chapter 7), but this has yet to be proven.

▶ Cerebral blood flow tends to increase in synchronized sleep, which may be explained by vasodilatation due to the hypoventilation-induced rise in $PaCO_2$ and by metabolic vasodilatation occurring in response to local increases in neuronal activity.

▶ During desynchronized sleep, there are large increases in cerebral blood flow in many regions of the fore-, mid- and hindbrain, where neurones are actively involved in the processes of sleep.

Reflexes during sleep

Intuitively, one might expect that reflex influences upon the cardiovascular and respiratory systems during sleep would be depressed. The available evidence indicates that such a view would be simplistic.

Cardiovascular reflexes

The first detailed studies on the role of the arterial baroreceptors and chemoreceptors during sleep were performed on the cat [1]. It was found that when the carotid sinus and aortic nerves had been sectioned, so denervating both carotid and aortic chemoreceptors, arterial pressure was moderately elevated during quiet wakefulness, fell to similar levels during synchronized sleep to those seen before denervation, but fell much more markedly during desynchronized sleep to levels well below those recorded in the intact animal. There was also an

increase in blood pressure variability at all times, but particularly during desynchronized sleep. This indicated that the baroreceptors or chemoreceptors were important in limiting the fall in arterial pressure during desynchronized sleep and in buffering the blood pressure variations.

A later study by the same group showed that after sino-aortic denervation the fall in total peripheral vascular conductance during desynchronized sleep was much greater. This could be attributed not only to greater splanchnic vasodilatation, but also to dilatation in the hindlimb. In other words, the muscle vasoconstriction that normally occurred during desynchronized sleep (see above) was reversed in direction. It was concluded that activity in the sino-aortic afferents buffers a central inhibitory influence of sleep upon both splanchnic and muscle sympathetic activity, so that its removal allowed the central inhibitory influence to dominate in both vascular beds. The explanation given for the vasoconstriction that normally occurs in muscle during desynchronized sleep was that it is due to a spinal reflex (see below and Fig. 7, later) and it was proposed that after sino-aortic denervation this spinal reflex was also overcome by the central inhibitory influence. These observations contrast markedly with the finding of Futuro-Neto and Coote [5], that a pattern of decreased sympathetic activity to kidney and splanchnic regions and increased sympathetic activity to muscle could still be recorded in the desynchronized sleep-like state seen in decerebrate cats, after sino-aortic denervation. These results suggested that this whole pattern of sympathetic activity was centrally generated, rather than being dependent on input from the sino-aortic afferents (for further discussion, see below and Fig. 9, later).

An interesting development of the work on intact cats was the finding that when the carotid baroreceptors and carotid chemoreceptors were selectively denervated during two separate operations, in animals in which aortic nerves had already been sectioned, enhancement of the fall in arterial pressure during the desynchronized sleep always occurred when the chemoreceptors were denervated, irrespective of the order of chemoreceptor and baroreceptor denervation [1] (see Fig. 8, later). These results strongly indicated that activity in the chemoreceptor afferent fibres plays a major role in limiting the fall in arterial pressure during desynchronized sleep, by exerting an excitatory influence upon sympathetic preganglionic neurones. An increase in peripheral chemoreceptor activity during desynchronized sleep could be explained by the increase in $PaCO_2$ and fall in PaO_2 (see above) and, secondly, by a decrease in tissue blood flow of the carotid body caused by the drop in arterial pressure.

Whether the chemoreceptors play a similar important role in regulating the fall in arterial pressure in other species has not been determined. However, it has been shown that in the rat the small rise in arterial pressure that usually occurs in this species during desynchronized sleep (see above) is converted, by sino-aortic denervation, to a substantial fall in arterial pressure [2]. This could be explained if the excitatory influence of the peripheral chemoreceptors upon sympathetic vasoconstrictor neurones is particularly strong in this species, a suggestion that is compatible with evidence that a tonic influence from the peripheral chemoreceptors plays a significant role in setting the normal level of arterial pressure in the rat.

Other studies have investigated the effects of changes in sino-aortic activity upon the cardiovascular system during sleep, rather than the role of their tonic activity. In the cat, the reflex rise in arterial pressure evoked by bilateral occlusion of the carotid arteries was much smaller during desynchronized sleep than during synchronized sleep [1], whereas in man the reflex bradycardia evoked by the pressor response to injection of phenylephrine (an α-adrenoreceptor agonist) was greater during desynchronized sleep than during wakefulness [2]. This might be taken to suggest that baroreceptor reflexes are oppositely affected in the two species. However, the reflex response to carotid occlusion was probably due mainly to baroreceptor unloading (rather than to effects on other receptor groups), and so the removal of baroreceptor-mediated inhibition of sympathetic preganglionic neurones would have to counteract the inhibitory effect of sleep on these neurones. By contrast, the baroreceptor-mediated excitation of cardiac vagal neurones and inhibition of cardiac sympathetic neurones evoked by phenylephrine would sum with the effect of sleep on these neurones. Thus it is not surprising that carotid occlusion was less effective than phenylephrine in producing a reflex response, and there is no reason to propose

either central inhibition, or facilitation, of the baroreceptor reflex during sleep. Nevertheless, from a practical point of view, these results suggest that any perturbation of arterial pressure that occurs during sleep is likely to be buffered more effectively if it is a rise, rather than a fall.

Respiratory reflexes

Reflex influences upon respiration deserve a brief mention in this chapter, to complement the material discussed above. The fact that $PaCO_2$ is increased during synchronized sleep, suggests that respiratory sensitivity to CO_2 may be altered [7,9]. In fact, the ventilatory response to hypercapnia undergoes two changes: (i) the position of the relationship between PCO_2 and ventilation shifts to higher PCO_2 levels and (ii) the sensitivity of the ventilatory response to CO_2 decreases (the slope $\Delta V/\Delta PCO_2$ decreases). There is also a much tighter relationship between $PaCO_2$ and ventilation than during wakefulness, i.e. the correlation coefficient is greater, indicating that ventilation is much more dependent on metabolic stimuli during synchronized sleep than during wakefulness.

Several studies have indicated that during desynchronized sleep, the sensitivity to CO_2 is greatly reduced relative to that seen in synchronized sleep (Fig. 5). However, when the tonic and phasic periods of desynchronized sleep are considered separately, it seems that during the tonic periods the sensitivity is the same as during synchronized sleep, whereas in the phasic periods there is virtually no sensitivity to CO_2 (Fig. 6). It is as if during phasic desynchronized sleep breathing is being driven by a central control system, which induces the rapid irregular breathing that is characteristic of this type of sleep, and the metabolic control by CO_2 is over-ridden [7,9].

Seen against this background, it is particularly remarkable that the respiratory responsiveness to changes in PaO_2 is preserved during sleep. In synchronized sleep, the correlation coefficient for the relationship between PaO_2 and ventilation is greater than during wakefulness, and the slope of the ventilation/PaO_2 relationship is only slightly decreased from that seen during wakefulness. During desynchronized sleep, the sensitivity to hypoxia is as great as during synchronized sleep (Fig. 5); the slope is not reduced during the phasic periods, although these periods are probably respon-

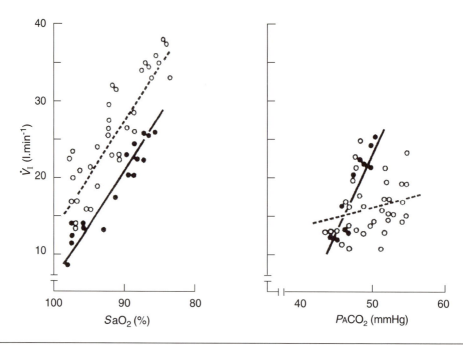

Fig. 5. Ventilatory responses to hypoxia and hypercapnia in the dog during synchronized and desynchronized sleep

$\dot{V}_I$ represents minute ventilation; SaO_2 indicates arterial saturation with oxygen; $PACO_2$ indicates partial pressure of carbon dioxide in alveolar gas; filled circles and continuous lines represent data obtained during synchronized sleep; open circles and dashed lines represent data obtained during desynchronized sleep. Reproduced with permission from Phillipson, E.A. (1977) Am. Rev. Respir. Dis. 115, 217–224

sible for the larger scatter of the data points (Fig. 5). Further, while the irregular pattern of breathing of desynchronized sleep persists during hypoxia, fluctuations in PaO_2 during desynchronized sleep have been shown to be considerably wider following sino-aortic denervation than in the intact state. Thus it seems that peripheral chemoreceptor activity normally limits the extent of the breathing irregularities during desynchronized sleep, probably in part by limiting apnoeas.

The significance of the preserved respiratory responsiveness to peripheral chemoreceptor activity is emphasized when one realizes that the respiratory responses to other afferent stimuli are generally reduced during sleep [7,9]. For example, the reflex response evoked by stimulation of slowly adapting lung-stretch receptors (Hering–Breuer reflex) persists during synchronized sleep, but is depressed during desynchronized sleep, the responses evoked by mechanical stimulation of the chest wall and by thermal stimuli are depressed or abolished dur-

ing both synchronized and desynchronized sleep, while stimulation of upper airway or broncho-pulmonary irritant receptors, which normally evokes coughing during wakefulness, can cause apnoea during all stages of sleep.

Thus the excitatory influence of the peripheral chemoreceptors upon respiration, which helps to prevent detrimental falls in PaO_2 during sleep, can be viewed as complementary to their excitatory influence upon sympathetic vasoconstrictor neurones, which helps to limit both the fall in arterial pressure and the arterial pressure variability associated with desynchronized sleep.

Importantly, the input from peripheral chemoreceptors can also induce arousal from sleep. In accord with other afferent stimuli which do this, such as hypercapnia, auditory stimuli, pulmonary irritant receptor stimulation, or somatic afferent stimulation, the threshold for arousal by chemoreceptors is increased in desynchronized sleep compared with synchronized sleep; in the dog, the arousal threshold increases from an arterial oxygen saturation of about 80–87% in synchronized sleep to 66–76% in desynchronized sleep [7,9]. Nevertheless, this still allows the peripheral chemoreceptors to produce the ultimate defence against hypoxia in sleep, in that arousal allows an appropriate behavioural response to the factor causing hypoxia, for example, to a pillow that is occluding nose and mouth, while the return to the awake state means that the respiratory sensitivity to hypoxia is improved.

▶ Apparent changes in the sensitivity of the arterial baroreceptor reflex during sleep may be explained by sleep-induced changes in the activity of sympathetic and cardiac vagal neurones. Similarly, respiratory reflexes are generally depressed in parallel with the reduced excitability of central respiratory neurones.

▶ The tonic input from peripheral chemoreceptors plays a major role in maintaining arterial pressure in tonic desynchronized sleep, and the reflex influence of peripheral chemoreceptors upon respiration is preserved in all stages of sleep.

▶ Stimulation of the peripheral chemoreceptors can readily cause arousal from sleep, which is of interest given that in the awake state they can activate the defence areas to produce the full pattern of the alerting response (see Chapter 3).

The role of the central nervous system

It is beyond the scope of this chapter to discuss the role of the central nervous system in initiating and maintaining the various stages of sleep. However, it is important to state here that sleep

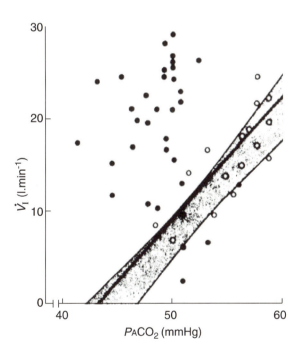

Fig. 6. **Ventilatory responses to hypercapnia during the phasic and tonic periods of desynchronized sleep**

$\dot{V}_I$ represents minute ventilation; $PACO_2$ indicates partial pressure of carbon dioxide in alveolar gas; shaded area represents 95% confidence limits of data obtained during synchronized sleep; open circles and solid line represent data and regression line (thick solid line) obtained during tonic periods of desynchronized sleep; filled circles represent data obtained during phasic periods of desynchronized sleep. Reproduced with permission from Sullivan, C.C., Murphy, E., Kozar, L.F. and Phillipson, E.A. (1979) J. Appl. Physiol. **47**, 17–25.

is not simply the passive effect of withdrawal of sensory inputs to the brain and the elimination of wakefulness, as was once thought.

Briefly, the waking state is generally considered to be maintained by tonic discharge from what is known as the ascending reticular formation, or reticular activating system of the brainstem and midbrain [3]. Synchronized sleep is associated with a decrease in this tonic discharge, but it is uncertain whether this is due to removal of an excitatory influence on the reticular neurones, or to active inhibition. There is also considerable evidence that desynchronized sleep is generated in the pontine reticular formation, in that rhythmic synchronous discharges occur in pontine neurones and trigger discharges in the lateral geniculate nucleus and occipital cortex. These are probably responsible for the eye movements of desynchronized sleep. However, the ascending influences that are responsible for EEG activation, the descending influences that are responsible for postural muscle hypotonic and the influences

responsible for the phasic events of desynchronized sleep are probably mediated by different groups of neurones within the brainstem. The discussion that follows is concerned only with a brief account of the role of the central nervous system in generating the cardiovascular and respiratory changes associated with sleep.

Cardiovascular changes
The cardiovascular changes associated with desynchronized sleep have attracted most attention. As is described above, during the tonic periods there is an increase in parasympathetic and decrease in sympathetic activity to the heart, a decrease in sympathetic activity to splanchnic and renal circulations, but an increase in sympathetic activity to muscle. Zanchetti and colleagues [1] concluded that the mechanisms responsible for the activation of sympathetic fibres to muscle are complicated. This is based on their finding that the vasoconstriction that occurs in the limb of cats during desynchronized sleep was abolished when the

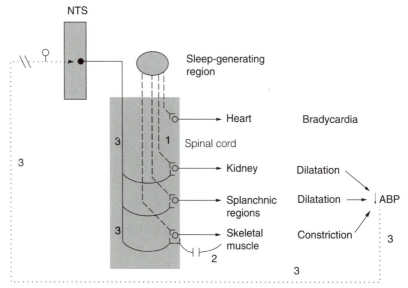

Fig. 7. Schematic diagram indicating how the nervous system may be involved in the cardiovascular changes that accompany desynchronized sleep

1, indicates influences from a central sleep-generating region on the sympathetic outflow to the heart and regional vascular beds; 2, indicates modification of that centrally generated influence upon the sympathetic outflow to skeletal muscle, by afferent input from skeletal muscle; 3, indicates the influence that the fall in arterial pressure which occurs during sleep exerts upon the sympathetic outflow via the sino-aortic afferent fibres (mainly chemoreceptors); continuous lines, indicate excitatory influences; dashed lines, indicate inhibitory influences. Abbreviations used: NTS, nucleus tractus solitarius; ABP, arterial blood pressure. This scheme is based on the work of Zanchetti et al. [1]. Breaks in pathways 2 and 3 indicate nerve sections that abolished vasoconstriction in skeletal muscle. For further explanation, see text.

dorsal roots that carry the afferent supply of the limb were cut (Fig. 7), and reversed to dilatation when the spinal cord was transected at L4, i.e. above the level of the dorsal root afferent input from the limb, but below the level of origin of the sympathetic output to the limb. They therefore proposed that the activation of the sympathetic fibres to the limbs was not dependent upon a descending influence from the brain, but rather on a reflex influence originating in the limbs themselves, which travels in the afferent somatic fibres and produces a spinal reflex in the sympathetic efferents (Fig. 7). This could be an excitatory reflex, in which case it would have to be proposed that there is a group of sensory receptors in the muscle that shows an increase in activity during desynchronized sleep and that the afferent input from these receptors leads to an increase in the sympathetic preganglionic activity to muscle. Alternatively, it could be an inhibitory reflex, in which case it would have to be proposed that there is a group

of receptors in muscle that is tonically active in the awake state, that these receptors have an inhibitory influence on sympathetic preganglionic activity to muscle and that they become less active when the muscle loses tone in desynchronized sleep. As is discussed above, this research group also found that sino-aortic denervation greatly accentuated the fall in arterial pressure and splanchnic vasodilatation that occurred during desynchronized sleep and reversed the hindlimb constriction to dilatation (Fig. 7) and that the fall in arterial pressure was also accentuated by specific denervation of the carotid chemoreceptors (Fig. 8). This led them to propose that the sino-aortic afferents, in particular the chemoreceptors, normally buffer a sleep-induced central inhibitory influence on both splanchnic and muscle vasoconstrictor tone, so that removal of their excitatory influence allowed the sympatho-inhibitory influence to predominate in muscle as well as splanchnic circulation.

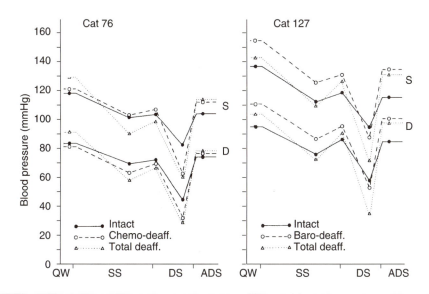

Fig. 8. Effect of selective denervation of carotid chemoreceptors (left) and of selective denervation of carotid baroreceptors (right) on changes in systolic (S) and diastolic (D) blood pressure during the wake-sleep cycle

(Left) cat with aortic nerves already cut, studied with sinus nerves intact (continuous line), then after selective denervation of carotid chemoreceptors (dashed line) and finally after denervation of carotid baroreceptors (dotted line). (Right) cat with aortic nerves already cut, studied with sinus nerves intact (continuous line), then after selective carotid baroreceptor denervation (dashed line) and finally after denervation of carotid chemoreceptors (dot-ted line). Abbreviations used: QW, quiet wakefulness; SS, synchronized sleep; DS, desynchronized sleep; ADS, after desynchronized sleep. Reproduced with permission from Zanchetti, A., Baccelli, G. and Mancia, G. (1973) In Hypertension: Mechanisms and Management (Onesti, G., Kim, K.E. and Moyer, J.H., eds.), pp. 133–140, Grune and Stratton, New York.

These results and proposals contrast markedly with those of Futuro-Neto and Coote [5], for in their decerebrate preparations of the cat which had undergone sino-aortic denervation, desynchronized sleep-like periods were accompanied by a decrease in sympathetic activity to heart, kidney and the splanchnic region, but an increase in muscle sympathetic activity. The increase in muscle sympathetic activity still occurred after paralysis, leading to the conclusion that it was not dependent on a reflex from skeletal muscle. However, it was greatly reduced by small lesions which cut the descending pathways in the spinal cord, indicating that it was dependent on descending influences from the brain. Electrical stimulation at different sites within the brainstem showed that there was a localized region of the caudal part of the nucleus raphe obscurus from which the full pattern of sympathetic activity recorded during the desynchronized sleep-like state could be evoked (Fig. 9). This indicated that the whole pattern of sympathetic activity, including the increase in muscle sympathetic activity, is generated as an entity, either within the nucleus raphe obscurus or by some pathway that runs through it.

It is difficult to reconcile these conflicting results. It should be noted that Zanchetti and colleagues inferred the direction of change in muscle sympathetic activity from limb vascular conductance. Thus it is possible that the various manoeuvres that affected the muscle vasoconstriction did not actually abolish the increase in muscle sympathetic activity. Rather, the muscle vasculature may have been dominated by a myogenic dilatation to the greater fall in arterial pressure seen after the various denervation procedures, such that this overcame a persisting influence of sympathetic excitation. It may also be noted that neither of the muscle-sympathetic reflexes required to explain their findings (see above) has been clearly demonstrated. On the other hand, the findings of Futuro-Neto and Coote are open to the criticism that, since they were obtained in a decerebrate preparation, removal of the excitatory and inhibitory influences of higher brain structures may have distorted the pattern of sympathetic activity recorded.

It seems agreed that the more generalized increases in sympathetic activity that characterize the phasic periods of desynchronized sleep are centrally generated. In intact cats the phasic

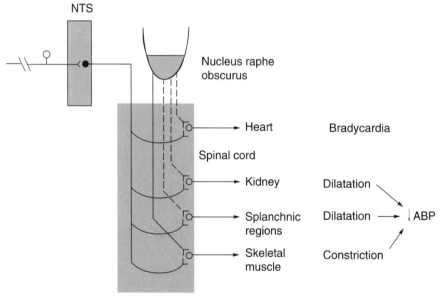

Fig. 9. Schematic diagram indicating how the nervous system may be involved in the cardiovascular changes that accompany desynchronized sleep

Continuous lines, indicate inhibitory influences; dashed lines, indicate excitatory influences. Abbreviations used: NTS, nucleus tractus solitarius; ABP, arterial blood pressure. This scheme is based on the work of Futuro-Neto and Coote [5,6]. The break in the afferent pathway to the NTS indicates that the experiments were performed after section of the sinus and aortic nerves. For further explanation, see text.

vasoconstrictions in limb muscle persisted after spinal cord transection below the sympathetic outflow and after deafferentiation of the limb, while experiments on the decerebrate cat which had been sino-aortically denervated revealed phasic bursts of sympathetic activity in cardiac, renal, splanchnic and muscle sympathetic fibres.

▶ The nervous mechanisms underlying the cardiac and peripheral vascular changes that accompany tonic desynchronized sleep have received most attention.

▶ The fall in heart rate can be attributed to increased cardiac vagal activity and decreased sympathetic activity. Simultaneously, there is a decrease in sympathetic activity to splanchnic and renal circulations and an increase in sympathetic activity to skeletal muscle.

▶ Evidence has been presented that the increase in sympathetic activity to muscle arises as a reflex response to a change in afferent activity from muscle. However, there is also evidence that the whole pattern of change in sympathetic activity is initiated by the caudal part of nucleus raphe obscurus.

Respiratory changes

It is apparent from the section above dealing with reflex regulation of respiration that the transitions from wakefulness to synchronized sleep to desynchronized sleep are accompanied by pronounced changes in the factors that dominate the control of breathing. Put simply, there are two major respiratory control systems that are separate but functionally integrated: the metabolic (or automatic) control system and the behavioural (or voluntary) control system (Fig. 10). The metabolic control system is primarily concerned with regulation of oxygen, carbon dioxide and hydrogen ion concentration, and depends upon inputs from central and peripheral chemoreceptors which are integrated with the chemoreceptor feedback from the lungs and chest wall: its output to the lower respiratory motor neurones in the spinal cord is via the ventrolateral spinal tracts. The behavioural control system can be attributed to cortical and forebrain structures and allows the respiratory system to be used for non-respiratory purposes: its output is via the corticospinal tracts.

During wakefulness, breathing is controlled by both systems, the metabolic system being dominant during quiet wakefulness and

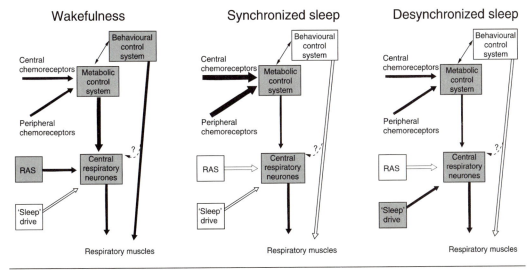

Fig. 10. **Diagrams illustrating the factors that determine breathing during wakefulness, synchronized and desynchronized sleep**

Shaded and unshaded boxes indicate components that are active and inactive, respectively; thickness of arrows gives qualitative indication of relative magnitudes of influences; open arrows indicate lack of influence; question marks indicate additional possible influence. Abbreviation used: RAS, reticular activating system. For further explanation, see text.

the behavioural system during more active wakefulness. But, in addition, there is a 'wakefulness drive' to respiration which apparently originates from the reticular activating system. During the transition from wakefulness to synchronized sleep there is not only a loss of the influence of behavioural system, but also of the wakefulness drive. This is illustrated by the fact that an unfortunate group of people with defective central chemoreceptors or damaged ventrolateral spinal tracts fail to breathe during synchronized sleep (Ondine's curse). In other words, the regular pattern that typifies synchronized sleep is under the dominant control of the metabolic system while the reduction in the responsiveness of respiration to afferent inputs (see above) is probably secondary to loss of the excitatory wakefulness drive to the respiratory neurones (Fig. 10). During desynchronized sleep the metabolic control system becomes less important, with the major exception of the input from peripheral chemoreceptors; breathing becomes dominated by a 'sleep drive' which is analogous to, but distinct from, the wakefulness drive (Fig. 10). This drive has been demonstrated by the observation that in the dog, progressive blockade of the major afferent inputs to respiration has little effect on breathing during desynchronized sleep: it seems to be related to the desynchronized sleep state itself. The episodes of more rapid, irregular breathing during desynchronized sleep that are temporally associated with the phasic periods of this stage of sleep seem to be dependent on another excitatory drive, which is analogous to that which is associated with behavioural activity in the awake state. The fact that the irregularities of breathing and the phasic non-respiratory events, such as ponto-geniculate-occipital discharges and rapid eye movements, occur synchronously, is consistent with the idea that they have a common brainstem origin.

▶ The respiratory changes that occur during synchronized sleep can be attributed to loss of a wakefulness drive to central respiratory neurones, while the irregular pattern of breathing in desynchronized sleep can be attributed to the predominating influence of a pattern generator within the pons and medulla. If, in the awake state, the defence areas of the brain exert a tonic influence upon the neurones of the rostral ventrolateral medulla which helps to maintain normal arterial pressure and respiration (see Chapter 3), then the fall in arterial pressure and respiration that accompany sleep may be attributable in part to loss of this 'alerting' drive.

Functional implications

The fall in cardiac output during synchronized sleep and the further fall during desynchronized sleep, which is combined with an increase in peripheral vascular conductance and fall in arterial pressure, decreases energy consumption, by decreasing the workload on the heart. The vasoconstriction in skeletal muscle in desynchronized sleep reduces blood flow to muscle, which becomes relatively inactive during sleep and helps to maintain arterial pressure. This, in turn, enables blood flow to be increased to metabolically active areas of the brain. The preserved influences of the peripheral chemoreceptors means that this can be achieved with little fall in PaO_2 and no significant reduction in the O_2 saturation of haemoglobin.

References
1. Mancia, G. and Zanchetti, A. (1980) Cardiovascular regulation during sleep. In Physiology in Sleep (Orem, J. and Barnes, C.D., eds.), pp. 1–55, Academic Press, New York
2. Coote, J.H. (1982) Respiratory and circulatory control during sleep. J. Exp. Biol. **100**, 223–244
3. Parmeggiani, P.L. and Morrison, A.R. (1990) Alterations in autonomic functions during sleep. In Central Regulation of Autonomic Function (Loewy, A.D. and Spyer, K.M., eds.), pp. 367–386, Oxford University Press, Oxford
4. Zbrozyna, A.W. and Westwood, D. (1988) Vascular changes in forearm and calf during sleep in man. Cardiovas. Res. **22**, 666–673
5. Futuro-Neto, H.A. and Coote, J.H. (1982) Changes in sympathetic activity to heart and blood vessels during desynchronized sleep. Brain Res. **252**, 259–268
6. Futuro-Neto, H.A. and Coote, J.H. (1982) Desynchronized sleep-like pattern of sympathetic activity elicited by electrical stimulation of sites in the brain stem. Brain Res. **252**, 269–276
7. Phillipson, E.A. and Bowes, G. (1986) Control of breathing during sleep. In Handbook of Physiology, Section III (Cherniack, N.S. and Widdicombe, J.G. eds.), pp. 642–689, Am. Physiol. Soc., Bethesda
8. Reveich, M., Isaacs, G., Evarts, E. and Kety, S.S. (1968) The effect of slow wave sleep and REM sleep on regional cerebral blood flow in cats. J. Neurochem. **15**, 301–306
9. Sullivan, C.E. (1980) Breathing in sleep. In Physiology in Sleep (Orem, J. and Barnes, C.D., eds.), pp. 213–272, Academic Press, New York

5

Regulation of blood volume

Roger Hainsworth and Mark J. Drinkhill
Academic Unit of Cardiovascular Studies, University of Leeds LS2 9JT, U.K.

Blood and body fluids

The 'typical' 70 kg man contains approximately 40 litres of water, which represents about 60% of his body weight. Of this volume, 25 litres is intracellular fluid and 15 litres is extracellular fluid (Fig. 1). Intracellular and extracellular fluids are separated by the cell membrane, which, although freely permeable to water, possesses several active and passive mechanisms which regulate the ions on either side of the membrane. The distribution of water is determined by osmotic forces exerted by the intracellular and extracellular ions. The extracellular fluid volume is particularly dependent on the quantity of sodium in the body and changes in, for example, the dietary intake of sodium may have an influence on blood volume. The other main boundary in relation to body water distribution is formed by the blood vessels, in particular the capillary membrane. Unlike the cell membrane, capillaries are freely permeable to electrolytes. However, they are virtually impermeable to plasma proteins, so that the division between plasma volume and the volume of the interstitial fluid is dependent on the balance between the hydrostatic and osmotic pressures on either sides of the capillary walls (see Chapter 8, Fig. 4). A dynamic equilibrium exists, with the outflow of fluid from capillaries to tissues being balanced by the inflow back into capillaries and that which is returned via the lymphatic system (see Chapter 8). Alterations in hydrostatic pressures change the flow of fluid. For example, in the upright position, interstitial fluid is absorbed from the upper part of the body and filtered into the tissues of the lower parts. Since, in humans, most of the body is below heart level, in the upright position there is a progressive net loss of blood volume. If a person stands upright and motionless (so that the 'muscle pump' mechanism is inoperative), plasma volume decreases by as much as 15% in half an hour. Loss of plasma volume is enhanced by arteriolar vasodilatation — for example, during body heating and exercise — and reduced by vasoconstriction. Thus it is important to recognize that plasma volume is not a static quantity, but that it represents the result of a dynamic equilibrium which can vary under physiological conditions.

> ▶ Blood volume is a dynamic quantity and depends on the balance of fluids between the vascular component and the intracellular fluids.
> ▶ This balance is dependent largely on the osmotic forces exerted by plasma proteins and electrolytes and the hydrostatic forces.

Blood volume

Under standard conditions, blood volume (plasma volume plus erythrocyte volume) is remarkably constant. On average, blood volume is about 80 ml/kg of body weight, or 5.5 litres for the 'average' man. A decrease in red cell volume, as in anaemia, is accompanied by a corresponding increase in plasma volume. The red cell volume is determined by the balance between red cell formation and red cell destruction. Assuming the cells are normal and healthy, their life-span is relatively constant. Production of red cells by the bone marrow is regulated by the hormone erythropoietin and can be increased in response to hypoxia. Changes in red cell numbers are normally slow, occurring over the course of days to weeks. Plasma volume, however, can be regulated much more quickly, both by changes in fluid input and by fluid loss.

There are two main sources of body water: ingestion of water, in liquids and foods, and metabolism, by oxidation of organic nutrients. Water is lost from the body through the skin, lungs, gastrointestinal tract and kidneys (Table 1). Although, in some circumstances, loss by extrarenal mechanisms can be very large, most of the fluid is usually excreted by the kidney. Fluid balance can be influenced by thirst, although in humans fluid input is more usually determined by social factors. The chief mechanism for regulating body fluid balance and, therefore, blood volume is by the kidney.

In this chapter, the pivotal role of the kidney in the regulation of blood volume is discussed. Another aspect in relation to blood volume is vascular capacitance and, since the bulk of blood volume is contained in veins, consideration is given to how venous pressures, distensibility and active venous constriction can influence the distribution of blood volume. Finally, the physiological responses associated with acute loss of blood volume are described.

Role of the kidney in regulation of blood volume

The content of sodium and water in the body is regulated mainly through the kidney. Sodium is particularly important, since it is the principal cation in the extracellular fluid. Sodium concentration largely determines extracellular fluid osmolality and so the body's content of sodium is closely related to extracellular fluid and plasma volume. In our 'average' man, the kidneys filter approximately 180 litres each day. Since the only source of this filtrate is the plasma, this means that the entire plasma volume is filtered some 60 times a day (Fig. 2). Clearly, quite small changes in the rate of filtration or reabsorption of salt and water by the kidney must have very large effects on the quantities retained by the plasma.

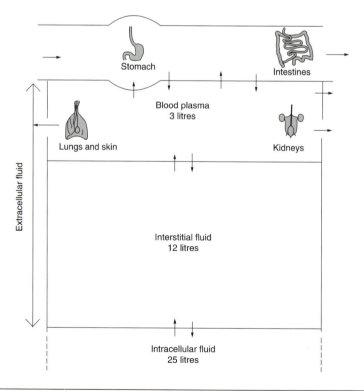

Fig. 1. **Body fluid compartments**
Note that water continuously crosses the boundaries of the various compartments, the equilibrium being determined largely by osmotic forces.

Table I. **Daily water balance**

Intake	ml per day
Drunk	1200
In food	1000
Metabolically produced	350
Total	2550

Output	ml per day
Insensible loss (skin/lungs)	900
Sweat	50
Faeces	100
Urine	1500
Total	2550

The average person usually excretes between 1 and 2 litres of urine per day, which means that 99% of the filtered water must have been reabsorbed. However, the rates of excretion of sodium and water can vary over an extremely wide range; for example, urinary water excretion can vary physiologically from approximately 0.4 litre/day to 25 litres/day.

Vasopressin (antidiuretic hormone, ADH)
The reabsorption of water is by osmosis and it depends upon the active reabsorption of sodium chloride. If the water permeability of the tubular epithelium is very high, water molecules are absorbed passively, almost as quickly as the actively transported sodium ions. The water permeability of the distal tubules and collecting ducts is subject to physiological control and the major determinant of this permeability is vasopressin. In the absence of vasopressin, the permeability of these segments is very low, while sodium reabsorption is able to occur as normal. Vasopressin is released into the blood from the posterior pituitary and its rate of release, and thus its plasma concentration, is largely controlled by osmoreceptors in the hypothalamus. The result of this mechanism is that a water load, which lowers the plasma osmolality, results in the inhibition of vasopressin and the consequent production of large volumes of dilute urine. The net effect is that the water load is excreted and plasma osmolality and extracellular fluid volumes are restored.

Renin–angiotensin–aldosterone system
Under the influence of a low renal arterial perfusion pressure, a low delivery of sodium chloride to the kidney or an increase in the renal sympathetic nerve activity, the juxtaglomerular cells lining the afferent arteriole secrete the hormone renin. Renin is a proteolytic enzyme which acts by cleaving a circulating plasma protein, angiotensinogen, into the 10-amino-acid peptide angiotensin I. This too is relatively inactive, but is cleaved further (by angiotensin-converting enzyme in the lung) to the highly active 8-amino-acid peptide, angiotensin II, which has a half-life of only 30 s. Angiotensin II is not only a very potent vasoconstrictor, but it also increases reabsorption of sodium by the proximal tubule and stimulates the release by the adrenal cortex of the potent, salt-retaining steroid, aldosterone. It also promotes the secretion of vasopressin from the posterior pituitary, resulting in water retention.

Adrenal cortical hormones
The hormones mainly concerned with the control of renal function are cortisol and aldosterone. These hormones act to reduce salt excretion by stimulating its reabsorption by the loop of Henle and the collecting duct. Aldosterone is 500 times more potent than cortisol in causing sodium retention. However, there is about 130 times more cortisol secreted and, therefore, its role in the control of sodium concentration should not be ignored.

Atrial natriuretic peptide
The existence of a humoral agent released by stretching of atrial myocytes was demonstrated by De Bold in 1979. Injections of atrial, but not ventricular, extracts were shown to cause pronounced natriuretic and diuretic responses. The active agent has now been identified, synthesized and shown to be a 28-amino-acid peptide which has been named as atrial natriuretic factor or atrial natriuretic peptide (ANP).

The physiological actions of ANP, in addition to causing diuresis and natriuresis by a direct effect on the kidney, are to cause vasodilatation, an increase in interstitial fluid volume and a decrease in renin release, and, thereby, a decrease in angiotensin and aldosterone production. It has also been suggested that ANP may augment cardiac afferent nerve activity and thereby promote reflex renal responses [1].

The stimulus for the release of ANP is atrial stretch, and does not involve neural pathways, although it has been suggested that the release of ANP may be modified by activity in

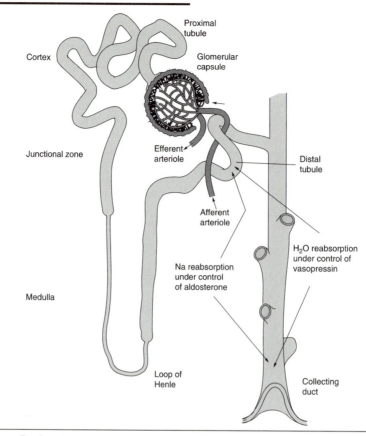

Fig. 2. A nephron
This diagram illustrates the sites of action of aldosterone and vasopressin.

efferent nerves and other humoral agents, including glucocorticoids, thyroid hormones and endothelin. However, these agents also have widespread actions on the cardiovascular system, so their direct effects on ANP release are uncertain.

The significance of ANP in the normal physiological control of blood volume is also uncertain. It is necessary to expand extracellular fluid volume by as much as 20% before there is an increase in the plasma level of ANP, and even then the response tends to be transient (5–15 min) in relation to the diuresis and natriuresis, which may last 3–4 h. More physiological interventions which increase atrial volumes, such as water immersion, do cause a 2–4-fold increase in plasma ANP. However, infusion of a similar quantity of exogenous ANP does not consistently result in either diuresis or natriuresis. It is likely that the net physiological effects of plasma volume expansion or atrial distension depend on many factors, of which ANP is only

one. Its physiological importance, therefore, has probably been overstated and its role still remains to be established [2].

Renal efferent nerves

The innervation of the kidney is by adrenergic sympathetic fibres. These innervate both afferent and efferent arterioles as well as the juxtaglomerular apparatus (Fig. 2). Increased activity in these nerves results in a decrease in glomerular filtration rate, and a consequent increase in the rate of reabsorption of sodium by the proximal renal tubule and the loop of Henle. In addition, increased activity in the renal efferent nerves directly increases sodium reabsorption by the proximal tubule, as well as activating the renin–angiotensin–aldosterone system. Thus an increase in renal nerve activity is one of the mechanisms available for promoting sodium retention and hence an increase in extracellular fluid and plasma volumes.

> ▶ The kidneys have a key role in blood volume regulation and retention of water and salt.
> ▶ They are under the influence of vasopressin and adrenalcortical hormones, particularly aldosterone.
> ▶ Increased activity in efferent renal nerves will promote plasma volume expansion.
> ▶ Control of vasopressin is largely effected through hypothalamic osmoreceptors; atrial receptors also have a role.

Reflex control of blood volume

Short-term regulation of arterial blood pressure is effected largely by the arterial baroreceptors. A fall in arterial pressure, which unloads baroreceptors, results in reflex vasoconstriction throughout the body, including the kidney. It is also associated with an increased secretion of vasopressin. Thus the effect is to cause salt and water retention and to increase blood volume. However, although it can be shown that baroreceptors can influence blood volume, they are unlikely to have an important role in its normal regulation. A moderate change in circulating blood volume does not greatly change the discharge frequency of the baroreceptors. It does, however, cause a relatively large change in central venous pressure and, consequently, in right and left atrial pressures. The great veins and atria, therefore, are ideally placed to sense changes in blood volume and play a pivotal role in the regulation of an individual's blood volume.

Atrial receptors
The heart, including the atria and adjoining great veins, is the origin of afferent fibres which travel in both parasympathetic and sympathetic nerves; both myelinated and non-myelinated fibres are involved.

Afferent nerves running in the sympathetic division — both myelinated and non-myelinated — enter the central nervous system through the spinal cord. Frequently they are connected to more than one sensory area which may not even be located in the same cardiac chamber. No specific receptor ending has been described, but discharge may be evoked in response to either mechanical events or chemical stimuli, such as bradykinin released by ischaemic myocardium, or both. It is difficult to ascribe a specific physiological role for these nerves, particularly in view of their diffuse distribution, although some may function as nociceptors and be responsible for the cardiac pain experienced during myocardial ischaemia.

Much more is known concerning the vagal innervation of the atria. There are many more non-myelinated afferent fibres (conduction velocity less than 2.5 m/s) than myelinated afferents. However, it is only the myelinated atrial afferents that are known to be attached to specific receptor terminals. Histological examination of the atria has revealed that these receptors are located in the endocardium of the heart and are localized mainly at the junctional regions of the superior and inferior venae cavae and right atrium and the pulmonary vein–left atrial junctions (Fig. 3); however, receptors have also been observed in the atrial walls and the appendages. Histologically, atrial receptors are described as complex, unencapsulated endings (Fig. 4). The diameter of the endings is 50–150 μm and there are approximately twice as many endings in the left atrium as in the right. The only other histological structure in the atrial wall which is thought to be of nervous origin is an endocardial end-net of branching strands. The origin and function of these fibres is uncertain.

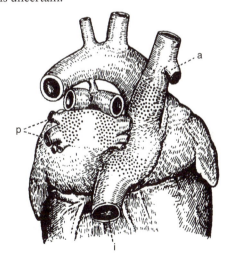

Fig. 3. Posterior view of the heart of a kitten showing the location of atrial receptors (dots)
Abbreviations used: a, azygos vein; p, pulmonary veins; i, inferior vena cava. Reproduced with permission from [15].

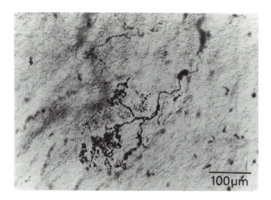

Fig 4. A complex unencapsulated atrial receptor

Photomicrograph prepared by Dr D.A.S.G. Mary

The discharge in myelinated afferents from atrial receptors can have one of three discharge patterns [3]: type A, which is synchronous with atrial systole ('a' wave); type B, which occurs during maximal atrial distension ('v' wave); and intermediate, which has both A and B discharge characteristics (Fig. 5). These discharge patterns, however, do not signify different receptor structures, since the type of discharge may be related to their position on the atrial wall: type A fibres may be excited when vigorous atrial contraction pulls on the vein–atrial junctions. The discharge characteristics can be changed by sympathetic stimulation, haemorrhage and infusions.

Relation between atrial receptor discharge and atrial pressure and volume

Atrial receptors are not blood volume receptors; they are distension receptors which sense atrial pressure and/or volume. Obviously, a change in blood volume is one of the factors influencing atrial receptor activity. There is a very good linear relationship between receptor activity and mean atrial pressure which can be varied by altering blood volume (Fig. 6).

The discharge of atrial receptors can also be influenced by long-term changes in blood volume. In one study, dogs were fed either a high- or a low-salt diet to result in a high or low blood volume, respectively [4]. There was no difference in the atrial pressures in the two groups of dogs, but the dogs with the higher blood volume had a higher atrial receptor discharge and a greater sensitivity of the discharge to changes in atrial pressure (Fig. 7).

Atrial receptors and urine flow

Experimentally, in animals, atrial receptor discharge can be increased either by distension of small balloons at the vein–atrial junctions, or, for the left atrium, by distension of a balloon to obstruct partially the mitral orifice. The reflex cardiovascular response is an increase in heart rate, mediated by the efferent sympathetic nerves [5], an effect which forms the basis of the 'Bainbridge reflex'. Studies of patterns of efferent sympathetic nerve activity in response to atrial distension show an increased discharge in

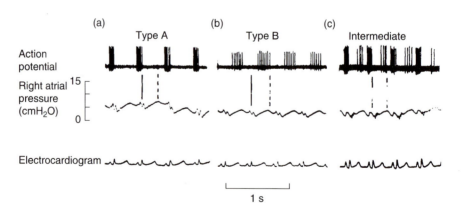

Fig. 5. Discharge activity in three atrial receptors
Traces of action potentials, right atrial pressure and electrocardiogram. (a) Type A discharge with high-frequency activity corresponding to 'a' wave of atrial pressure; (b) type B discharges relating to atrial pressure 'v' wave; (c) intermediate discharge with both type A and B characteristics. Reproduced with permission from [16].

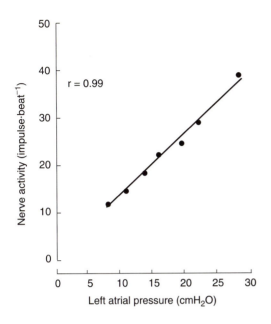

Fig. 6. **The relationship between activity in a single left atrial fibre and mean left atrial pressure**
Reproduced with permission from [3].

effect which is mediated through the renal nerves, and to decrease plasma cortisol activity [9]. Both these actions, as already explained, would promote salt and water excretion.

It has also been suggested that a specific diuretic substance may be involved in the response. This is a substance which is dependent on the integrity of the vagus nerves and persists after ablation of the pituitary gland and adjacent hypothalamus. Its identity, however, remains unknown and its physiological significance has not, as yet, been established.

Atrial receptors in humans
Almost all the precise information on the effects of stimulation of atrial receptors is based on experiments using animals, mainly anaesthetized dogs. In man, attempts have been made to produce situations which would be expected to alter atrial receptor discharge, using proce-

the cardiac nerves, no change in the lumbar or splenic nerves and a decrease in efferent renal nerve discharge [6].

It has been known for nearly 40 years that atrial distension results in an increase in urine flow. The involvement of atrial receptors in this response was shown by use of a discrete atrial stimulus and by preventing the response by cooling the vagus nerves to temperatures which block the increase in discharge in myelinated afferent fibres (Fig. 8). Less clear has been the efferent mechanism responsible for the change in the urine flow. The decrease in efferent renal nerve discharge and haemodynamic consequences of the reflex increase in heart rate result in an increase in salt as well as in water excretion. Pharmacological blockade of efferent autonomic mechanisms or use of a neurally isolated kidney, however, does not prevent the diuretic response, which must therefore be mediated, at least partly, through one or more blood-borne agents. It has been shown that atrial receptor stimulation inhibits vasopressin release from the pituitary gland and this can, at least partly, explain the diuretic response [7].

Stimulation of atrial receptors has also been shown to decrease renin release [8], an

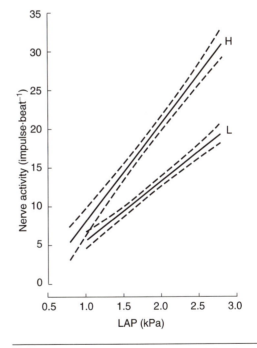

Fig. 7. **The relationship between activity from left atrial receptors and atrial pressure (LAP) in a group of dogs fed a low-salt diet to induce a low blood volume (L), and a group on a high-salt diet resulting in a high blood volume (H)**
Note the increased sensitivity of the atrial receptors in the high-salt group. Reproduced with permission from [4].

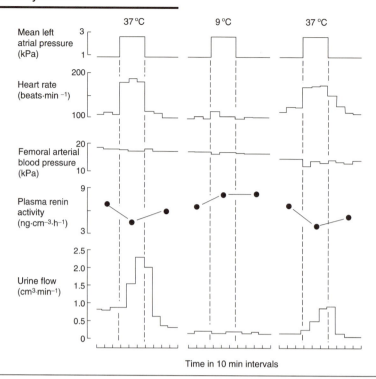

Fig. 8. Responses in one dog to left atrial distension with the cervical vagus nerves at body temperature (left and right panels) and cooled to 9°C to block the increase in neural activity in myelinated afferent fibres

Traces, from top, show mean left atrial pressure, heart rate, femoral arterial blood pressure, plasma renin activity and urine flow. Note that with the vagi at body temperature, atrial distension causes tachycardia, no change in arterial pressure, a decrease in plasma renin activity and an increase in urine flow. With the increase in neural activity in myelinated vagal afferent fibres blocked, all the responses to atrial distension were prevented. Reproduced with permission from [8].

dures which include head-down tilt, saline infusions and body immersion. These procedures have not been shown to decrease vasopressin levels and, generally, results obtained with humans have been disappointingly inconsistent [10,11]. This inconsistency probably reflects the difficulty in applying a discrete stimulus to atrial receptors, and any effects are likely to be the result of changes in the stimuli to many disparate receptor populations.

▶ Atrial receptors situated at the great vein–atrial junctions are stimulated by atrial distension, which in turn is influenced by, among other things, blood volume.
▶ Volume expansion results in reflex inhibition of vasopressin, renin and, therefore, angiotensin and aldosterone; it also results in a reduction in efferent renal nerve activity.

▶ All these effects promote salt and water excretion.
▶ Although these responses have been demonstrated experimentally in animal preparations, their importance in the control of blood volume, particularly in people, remains unclear.

Vascular capacitance

The volume of blood contained within a region of the circulation is determined partly by passive influences, which depend on the distensibility of the vessels and on extravascular forces, and partly on the degree of active vasoconstriction of the vascular smooth muscle. Since about 70% of the blood is contained in veins, these vessels are considered to be the body's capacitance vessels, and factors which influence the volume of blood in the veins are of importance in determination of the distribution of blood within the body.

Compliance is the change in volume in a region or a vessel per unit change in pressure, i.e. the slope of the volume–pressure relationship. It is not the same as capacitance, which is the actual volume contained at a given distending pressure. Compliance is dependent on the degree of filling and the distensibility of the blood vessels, mainly veins. For the whole body, compliance is about 2.5 ml/kg of body weight for every 1 mmHg change in venous pressure. This implies that for a 70 kg man a change in blood volume of 1 litre would be accompanied by a change in central venous pressure of a little over 5 mmHg. This change in pressure, although small, would activate the mechanisms associated with the control of blood volume which have been described above.

The high compliance of veins results in venous volume being partly dependent on blood flow and, thus, indirectly affected by the state of arteriolar constriction. The mechanism of this is that an increase in blood flow to a region causes an increase in pressure, particularly in small veins and venules, and, therefore, an increase in regional blood volume. Conversely, arteriolar constriction results in a decrease in flow and passive relaxation of the smaller veins.

It is important to remember that it is not actually the pressure within a vein that is related to its volume but rather the transmural pressure. This is particularly important in the legs, where the force exerted by the skeletal muscle on veins, the 'muscle pump', can empty veins despite a high intravascular pressure. This effect is also relevant in the splanchnic circulation; this region is highly distensible and contributes as much as half of the whole body's compliance. When the average man is standing, the effect of gravity is to increase pressure in the abdominal veins to about 20 mmHg; if this were the distending pressure it would result in accumulation of nearly 2 litres of blood. However, the abdominal viscera are effectively contained within a rigid bag (the abdomen) and the force exerted by the weight of the viscera greatly reduces the transmural venous pressures.

The other important influence on regional blood volume is the vascular capacitance. This is dependent on the state of constriction of the vascular smooth muscle. Capacitance and compliance may change in opposite ways. For example, in a distended vein, the volume is little affected by a change in pressure and so the compliance is low; however, when the vein is stimulated to constrict, this reduces its capacitance but, because it is no longer fully distended, its compliance is increased.

Active capacitance responses can be studied only with the use of carefully controlled preparations in which the region investigated is vascularly isolated, the inflow of blood is controlled and venous pressure is held constant. Under these conditions, any change in blood volume in the region represents a change in capacitance. There have been many studies of capacitance in the circulation of the limb. Indeed, in humans, limbs are the only regions in which it is possible to investigate capacitance responses. Although the limb vascular volume varies with changes in its arterial inflow, these changes simply reflect what would be expected because of the vascular compliance. There is no evidence of any active capacitance changes in that circulation. This implies that the veins draining muscle and skin essentially function only as blood conduits. In fact, owing to the very high flow through these regions during physical exercise or heat load, any significant venoconstriction would be more likely to impede the return of blood to the heart than to enhance it.

The situation in the abdominal vascular bed, however, is quite different. Splanchnic blood volume is relatively large (about 25% of blood volume) and, under conditions of stress, activity in efferent sympathetic nerves would reduce blood flow. Measured under conditions of constant blood flow, it has been shown that stimulation of the splanchnic sympathetic nerves in the dog can mobilize about 7.5 ml of blood per kg of body weight [12]. Splanchnic capacitance vessels have been shown to be highly sensitive to low levels of sympathetic efferent nervous activity. Stimulation of the splanchnic nerves at only 1 impulse/s results in expulsion of nearly half the maximum possible change. At 2 impulse/s, two-thirds of the maximal change is expelled. Changes in vascular resistance at these low stimulus frequencies are relatively small (Fig. 9).

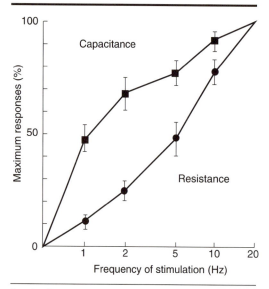

Fig. 9. Responses of splanchnic vascular resistance (●) and capacitance (■) to graded stimulation of efferent splanchnic sympathetic nerves

Results given as means ± S.E.M. from 10 dogs and the responses at each stimulus frequency are expressed as a percentage of that at 20 Hz. This shows that at stimulus frequencies of 1 and 2 Hz, capacitance responses are much greater proportions of maximal than are the corresponding resistance responses. Reproduced with permission from [12].

The splanchnic capacitance vessels also participate in cardiovascular reflexes and have been shown to constrict in response to various stimuli, including unloading of carotid and aortic baroreceptors and stimulation of peripheral and central chemoreceptors. They dilate in response to chemical stimulation of cardiac receptors. The high sensitivity of splanchnic capacitance vessels to low levels of sympathetic efferent activity (Fig. 9) also explains why a gradual decrease in carotid baroreceptor pressure first results predominantly in capacitance responses and only induces large resistance changes when carotid sinus pressure decreases to levels approaching the baroreceptor threshold.

Because of the impossibility of making adequate assessments of capacitance in humans, any quantitative assessments of their role is based on extrapolation from animal studies. The maximum capacitance response to direct or reflex stimulation of sympathetic nerves in dogs is about 7.5 ml/kg of body weight. However, about one-third of that response is due to contraction of the spleen, which is comparatively a

very large organ in the dog and small in people. Therefore, assuming that people behave like a dog without a spleen, the maximum possible change in capacitance would be of the order of 5 ml/kg of body weight. If people, like dogs, have a very high sensitivity of vascular capacitance to low levels of sympathetic activity, it is likely that a relatively modest cardiovascular stress would 'use up' most of the capacitance response, leaving little further 'reserve'. However, as was pointed out above, vascular volume is also dependent on blood flow, so arteriolar constriction would also result in passive capacitance changes and these could be of a magnitude similar to those resulting from active changes in capacitance.

During motionless standing, the dependent veins distend due to gravitational stress (Fig. 10), central venous pressure falls and cardiac output typically falls by about 20%. Arterial blood pressure, however, is normally well-maintained by reflex mechanisms which include constriction of the arteriolar resistance vessels. Constriction of capacitance vessels is also likely to make an important contribution by limiting the amount of venous distension and, thereby, reducing the fall in cardiac filling pressure. In the absence of such a response, the postural fall in cardiac output would be likely to be considerably greater and the incidence of posturally induced hypotension when people stand up would be much greater.

▶ Capacitance vessels are considered to be veins and venules, as they contain most of the blood volume and, due to their high compliance, they can adjust to changes in volume with only a small pressure change.
▶ Capacitance of veins is actively regulated by the vascular smooth muscle, but passive volume changes are of similar magnitude and can be effected by changes in the blood flow causing changes in distending pressure.
▶ Only the splanchnic circulation has been shown to have an active capacitance role. It is under control of sympathetic noradrenergic nerves and is particularly sensitive to low levels of sympathetic activity.
▶ Reflexes which control sympathetic nervous activity, including baroreceptors, chemoreceptors and cardiac receptors, also control vascular capacitance.

> ▶ The effect of a decrease in capacitance is to limit venous distensibility and to enhance return of blood to the heart. In man this mechanism is likely to be of particular importance in the adjustment of the cardiovascular system to the upright posture.

Haemorrhage

Haemorrhage refers to the loss of whole blood from the body; however, the physiological

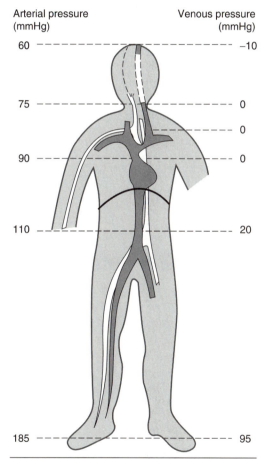

Arterial pressure (mmHg)   Venous pressure (mmHg)

60	–10
75	0
	0
90	0
110	20
185	95

Fig. 10. **Effects of gravity on arterial and venous pressures at different levels in upright man**

Below the heart, both pressures increase, resulting in venous distension and an increase in tissue fluid formation. Above the heart, pressures decrease and the brain is particularly susceptible to low arterial blood pressures.

effects are essentially those of a decrease in circulating blood volume. Thus similar effects occur in hypovolaemia due to dehydration or burn injury. In addition, prolonged standing, particularly in hot environments, can result in similar changes, owing to the combination of distension of capacitance vessels below heart level (venous pooling) and filtration of capillary fluid. Experimentally, the effects of haemorrhage can also be simulated by passive head-up tilting and by the application of a subatmospheric pressure to the lower body which distends veins and increases tissue fluid formation.

The responses to haemorrhage fall into two distinct phases [13]. In phase I, which is the response to the loss of up to about 20% of blood volume, arterial blood pressure is remarkably well-maintained, despite a fall in cardiac output. In phase II, which typically ensues when about 25–35% of blood volume has been lost, blood pressure abruptly falls and the subject loses consciousness. Much of what we know concerning the effects of haemorrhage emanates from studies carried out during the Second World War. However, although much research has been carried out since, we still do not fully understand all the mechanisms responsible.

Phase I: non-hypotensive haemorrhage
Progressive blood loss results in decreases in central venous pressure and cardiac output which are linearly related to the volume lost. The fact that cardiac output is decreased while heart rate is increased by reflex mechanisms means that the cardiac stroke volume must be considerably reduced. Stroke volume is the major determinant of arterial pulse pressure, and the decrease in stroke volume explains the reduction of pulse pressure. Despite the marked reduction in cardiac output, mean arterial blood pressure remains very little changed.

The effector mechanisms responsible for maintaining blood pressure in the face of a decrease in blood flow are well-understood. The main response is a constriction of arterioles and a consequent increase in vascular resistance, which is accompanied by capacitance vessel constriction. There is also an increase in heart rate, but, in the situation where cardiac filling pressure is low, the increase in rate is largely offset by a decrease in stroke volume, so that this has little effect on the cardiac output. The increase in vascular resistance has been demonstrated by measurements in the forearm by plethysmography. Assessments of total peripheral vascular resistance and of resistance in various other vascular beds have shown the vasoconstriction to be widespread. In people, recordings have been made from peripheral sympathetic nerves and simulated haemorrhage has been shown to increase such sympathetic activity. In addition to neurally mediated vasoconstriction, haemorrhage has also been shown to increase the concentrations in the blood of several vasoactive hormones including adrenaline, noradrenaline and angiotensin. Although there is agreement concerning the efferent mechanisms which maintain blood pressure during moderate haemorrhage the same cannot be said for afferent mechanisms. Arterial baroreceptors undoubtedly play a key role, particularly when there is a fall in arterial pressure. Even in the absence of a change in mean pressure, a decrease in the arterial pulse pressure would provide the necessary signal to elicit vasoconstriction.

There have been a number of claims that low-pressure 'cardiopulmonary' receptors may play an important role in initiating the responses to mild to moderate haemorrhage. During low levels of lower body suction, which simulates mild blood loss, it has been possible to demonstrate an increase in vascular resistance in the absence of any change in mean arterial pressure and even with little change in pulse pressure. Thus it was thought unlikely that the activity of the arterial baroreceptors was altered. The main change has been a fall in central venous and atrial pressures. The problem with this line of reasoning is that the so-called 'cardiopulmonary' receptors are not a homogeneous group. They are situated in many diverse regions, including atria, ventricles, pulmonary arteries and lungs, and changes in the activity of these different groups of receptors may result in differing reflex responses. Furthermore, none of the reflexes has been shown, convincingly, to be capable of causing the appropriate responses to mild haemorrhage. Another important point is that in animal studies in which the arterial baroreceptors were denervated, haemorrhage failed to cause an increase in vascular resistance, and this suggests a dominant role for the baroreceptors [14]. It seems likely, therefore, that arterial baroreceptors are the principal and perhaps the only mechanism responsible for the increase in vascular resistance occurring in response to haemorrhage.

Phase II: hypotensive haemorrhage

A more severe depletion of circulating blood volume, particularly when it occurs suddenly, results in the sudden failure of the compensatory mechanisms and an abrupt fall in arterial pressure and, frequently, also of heart rate (Fig. 11) This is the vasovagal syncope, so called by Sir Thomas Lewis because its characteristic features are a fall in vascular resistance and, usually less importantly, a vagally induced bradycardia. Hypotensive haemorrhage is not the same as irreversible shock (see below). A comparable response may occur during standing, particularly when standing motionless in a hot environment, due to reduction in the return of blood to the heart. The mechanism responsible for switching suddenly from the normal compensatory responses of vasoconstriction and tachycardia to vasodilatation and bradycardia, has been the subject of much speculation but still remains unknown.

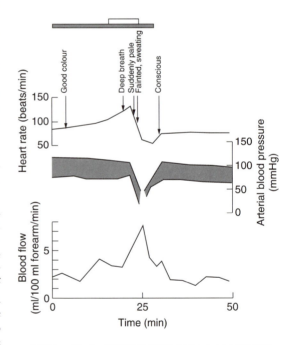

Fig. 11. **Effects of haemorrhage in a normal subject**
Shaded bar indicates venous return impeded by application of tourniquets to both thighs; open bar indicates venesection. Note that initially mean blood pressure was well maintained and heart rate increased. Suddenly, both blood pressure and heart rate fall. This is accompanied by an increase in forearm flow, signifying intense vasodilatation. Reproduced with permission from [17].

The characteristic feature of the phase II reaction is a decrease in vascular resistance. Recordings of efferent sympathetic discharge in some people who fainted revealed an abrupt cessation of all activity. There is no evidence of an increase in activity in vasodilator nerves. Indeed, in primates (including humans), there is little evidence even for the existence of vasodilator nerves (see Chapter 3). The abrupt cessation of vasoconstrictor activity after intense vasoconstriction is likely to be accompanied by vasodilation due to accumulation of vasodilator metabolites (see Chapter 7).

The vasovagal reaction is widely known to be accompanied by bradycardia. The bradycardia can occasionally amount to a period of complete asystole lasting for up to 30 s, but usually amounts to only a reduction in heart rate, to lit-tle less than normal resting values. The bradycardia, however, usually follows rather than precedes the hypotension. Usually, it makes lit-tle or no contribution to the hypotension, and the use of cardiac pacemakers to maintain con-stant heart rates during simulated haemorrhage (head-up tilting or application of lower-body negative pressure) does not have any influence on the time to onset of phase II. From a clinical point of view, the most significant aspect of the bradycardia is that the failure to observe a tachycardia in a bleeding patient does not nec-essarily imply the absence of severe haemor-rhage or shock: they may already be in phase II.

Hypotensive haemorrhage is also associ-ated with quite marked changes in the blood concentrations of vasoactive hormones (Fig. 12). The sharp rise in adrenaline and fall in

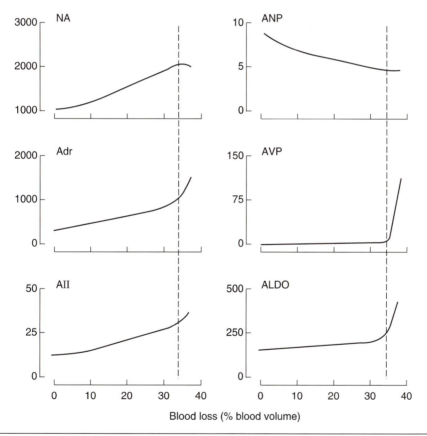

Fig. 12. Schematic diagram to show changes in some plasma hor-mone levels in response to graded blood loss

Dotted line indicates the onset of Phase II. All units are in pmol/l. Abbreviations used: NA, noradrenaline; Adr, adrenaline; AVP, vasopressin, AII, angiotensin II, ANP, atrial natriuretic peptide; ALDO, aldosterone. Adapted with permission from Ludbrook (1993).

noradrenaline levels may contribute to the vasodilatation. Phase II is also associated with increases in plasma levels of angiotensin II and vasopressin, and it is conceivable that during prolonged hypotensive haemorrhage these hormones may help to raise arterial pressure by causing vasoconstriction.

The trigger that suddenly changes the apparently appropriate response of vasoconstriction (Phase I) to the apparently inappropriate one of vasodilatation (Phase II) is unknown. Most reflexes function as negative feed-back mechanisms, so that a decrease in blood pressure would be expected to lead to responses which at least partly correct the disturbance. What appears to happen in hypotensive haemorrhage is that a fall in blood pressure triggers a mechanism which causes blood pressure to fall further and precipitously and to lead to loss of consciousness. One theory which has gained popularity is that the hypotensive response occurs as the result of stimulation of cardiac ventricular receptors. The postulated mechanism is that, when cardiac filling is greatly impaired and the cardiac sympathetic drive enhanced, the powerful contraction of the nearly empty ventricle stimulates afferent activity in the non-myelinated nerves. Some support for this theory comes from observations of an increase in activity in one particular group of cardiac afferent fibres in the cat during haemorrhage, those identified as originating in the ventricles. However, this occurred in only a minority of fibres studied; the discharge rate of most of the fibres actually decreased. Furthermore, in animals, cardiac denervation does not consistently influence the development of vasodilatation in response to haemorrhage. In addition, observations in humans also seem to cast doubt on the ventricular receptor theory since the response has been observed following heart transplant, when the ventricles of the transplanted heart have no sensory innervation. It is, therefore, likely that more than one triggering factor is involved.

It seems probable that central nervous mechanisms are involved. In particular, in animals opioids may be implicated because antagonists have been shown to prevent the onset of vasodilatation. There have been no adequate studies, however, in humans, and the mechanism which is responsible for the sudden onset of a seemingly inappropriate vasodilatation remains one of physiology's intriguing mysteries.

'Irreversible shock'

The older literature classified the effects of severe haemorrhage into reversible and irreversible shock. Reversible shock implied that, following replacement of the blood, the patient recovered. In irreversible shock, transfusion of blood did not restore the blood pressure and the patient would die. Irreversible shock due solely to haemorrhage rarely, if ever, occurs. Severe and prolonged haemorrhagic shock is frequently associated with tissue trauma and this is likely to result in septicaemia and endotoxaemia. The combination of this with underperfusion of tissues results in several potentially fatal consequences including acidosis, renal and hepatic failure, pulmonary hypertension, cardiac failure and disseminated intravascular coagulation.

The mechanisms for causing the changes in endotoxaemic shock are the subject of intensive research. A variety of cytokines, including tumour necrosis factor, interleukins, interferons and platelet-activating factor, are involved. A detailed review of the changes in septic shock, however, is outside the scope of this chapter.

▶ There are two types of cardiovascular response to haemorrhage.

▶ Non-hypotensive haemorrhage: moderate blood loss.

— Increased sympathetic activity to blood vessels and heart prevents a fall in mean arterial pressure.

— The stimulus to this response is decreased baroreceptor input, due to the fall in arterial pulse pressure.

— A role for low-pressure intrathoracic receptors has been proposed but not proven.

▶ Hypotensive haemorrhage: more severe blood loss leads to a sudden fall in pressure and imminent or actual unconsciousness.

— Associated with abrupt cessation of sympathetic activity and consequent vasodilatation.

— Heart rate is slower than during the non-hypotensive haemorrhage and occasionally there may be pronounced bradycardia.

— This phase of haemorrhage is accompanied by humoral changes including increases in plasma adrenaline and decreases in noradrenaline.

— The trigger responsible for initiating this response is unknown.

Suggestions for further reading

Blood volume control

Cowley, A.W. (1992) Long term control of arterial blood pressure. Physiol. Rev. **72**, 231–300

Hainsworth, R. (1991) Reflexes from the heart. Physiol. Rev. **71**, 617–657

Vascular capacitance

Hainsworth, R. (1986) Vascular capacitance: its control and importance. Rev. Physiol. Biochem. Pharmacol. **105**, 101–173

Hainsworth, R. (1990) The importance of vascular capacitance in cardiovascular control. News Physiol. Sci. **5**, 250–254

Haemorrhage

Hainsworth, R. (1992) Syncope and Fainting. In Autonomic Failure: A Textbook of Clinical Disorders of the Autonomic Nervous System, 3rd Edition (Bannister, R. and Mathias, C.J., eds.), pp. 761–781, Oxford University Press, Oxford

Ludbrook, J. (1993) Haemorrhage and Shock. In Reflex Control of the Cardiovascular System in Health and Disease (Hainsworth, R. and Mark, A.L., eds.), pp. 463–490, Saunders, London

References

1. Brenner, B.M., Ballerman, B.J., Gunning, M.E. and Zeidel, M.L. (1990) Diverse biological actions of atrial natriuretic peptide. Physiol. Rev. 70, 665–669

2. Goetz, K.L. (1990) Evidence that atriopeptin is not a physiological regulator of sodium excretion. Hypertension 15, 9–19

3. Mary, D.A.S.G. (1987) Electrophysiology of atrial receptors. In Cardiogenic Reflexes (Hainsworth, R., McWilliam, P.N. and Mary, D.A.S.G., eds.), pp. 3–17, Oxford University Press, Oxford

4. Hicks, M.N., Mary, D.A.S.G. and Walters, G.E. (1987) Atrial receptor discharge in dogs with chronically induced differences in blood volume. J. Physiol. 393, 491–497

5. Ledsome, J.R. and Linden, R.J. (1964) A reflex increase in heart rate from distension of the pulmonary vein–atrial junctions. J. Physiol. 170, 456–473

6. Karim, F., Kidd, C., Malpus, C.M. and Penna P.E. (1972) The effect of stimulation of the left atrial receptors on sympathetic efferent nerve activity. J. Physiol. 227, 243–260

7. Bennett, K.L., Linden, R.J. and Mary, D.A.S.G. (1984) The atrial receptors responsible for the decrease in plasma vasopressin caused by distension of the left atrium in the dog. Q. J. Exptl. Physiol. 69, 73-81

8. Drinkhill, M.J., Hicks, M.N., Mary, D.A.S.G. and Pearson, M.J. (1988) The effect of stimulation of the atrial receptors on plasma renin activity in the dog. J. Physiol. 398, 411–421

9. Drinkhill, M.J, and Mary, D.A.S.G. (1989) The effect of stimulation of the atrial receptors on plasma renin activity in the dog. J. Physiol. 413, 299–313

10. Goldsmith, S.R., Francis, G.S., Cowley, A.W. and Cohn, J.N. (1982) Response of vasopressin and norepinephrine to lower body negative pressure in humans. Am. J. Physiol. 243, H970–H973

11. Egan, B., Grekin, R., Ibsen, H., Osterziel, K. and Julius, S. (1984) Role of cardiopulmonary mechanoreceptors in ADH release in normal humans. Hypertension 6, 832–836

12. Karim, F. and Hainsworth, R. (1976) Responses of abdominal vascular capacitance to stimulation of splanchnic nerves. Am. J. Physiol. 231, 434–440

13. Shadt, J.C. and Ludbrook, J. (1991) Hemodynamic and neurohumoral responses to acute hypovolemia in conscious mammals. Am. J. Physiol. 260, H305–H318

14. Shadt, J.C. and Gaddis, R.R. (1986) Cardiovascular responses to hemorrhage and naloxone in conscious baro-denervated rabbits. Am. J. Physiol. 251, R909–R915

15. Nonidez, J.F. (1937) Identification of the receptor areas in the venae cavae and pulmonary veins which initiate reflex cardiac acceleration (Bainbridge's reflex). Am. J. Anat. 61, 203–231

16. Kappagoda C.T., Linden R.J. and Mary, D.A.S.G. (1976) Atrial receptors in the cat. J. Physiol. 262, 431–446

17. Barcroft, H. and Edholm, O.G. (1945) On the vasodilatation in human skeletal muscle during post-haemorrhagic fainting. J. Physiol. 104, 161–175

6

Cardiovascular responses to exercise: central and reflex contribution

John H. Coote
Department of Physiology, The Medical School, University of Birmingham, Birmingham B15 2TT, U.K.

Introduction

Humans are capable of quite astonishing physical achievements. For me, the completion of a 72-mile fell run of 44 peaks in under 24 hours involving 29000 ft of ascent in the English Lake District (Fig. 1), or perhaps the solo ascent of Everest without supplementary oxygen, are particularly noteworthy.

We are able to accomplish these feats only through a series of complex interactions within the body, involving nearly all of the body's systems. While the muscles perform the work, the heart and blood vessels deliver the nutrients and, with the help of the lungs, provide oxygen and remove carbon dioxide from the tissues. The nervous and endocrine systems integrate all of this activity into a meaningful performance. Practically no tissue or organ escapes involvement. Even the simplest movements involved in our everyday activities require a wide array of interaction.

Paramount in this response are the cardiovascular changes. During exercise, the cardiovascular system is challenged to supply the increased metabolic needs of the muscle, to dissipate heat and to maintain the requirements of other essential organs. To achieve this there is a repatterning of autonomic nerve activity which is indicated by the redistribution of blood flow to various organs (Fig. 2). Sympathetic nerve activity to the heart and blood vessels is increased, while the parasympathetic activity to the heart is decreased. Cardiac output increases some six times in very fit individuals and blood flow to skeletal muscle becomes a greater proportion of this by increasing to about 85% of cardiac output compared with 15% at rest (Fig. 2). The importance of these changes may perhaps best be appreciated by considering what would happen if they were absent during mild exercise requiring, for example, 1 litre of oxygen each minute. Assuming that, at rest, about 1 litre of the cardiac output goes to skeletal

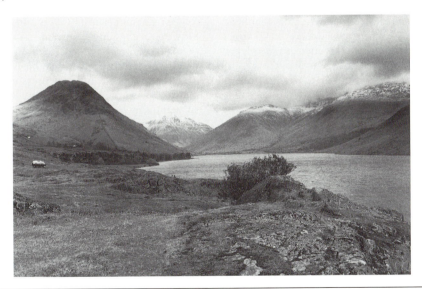

Fig. 1 **The English Lake District viewed from Wasdale**

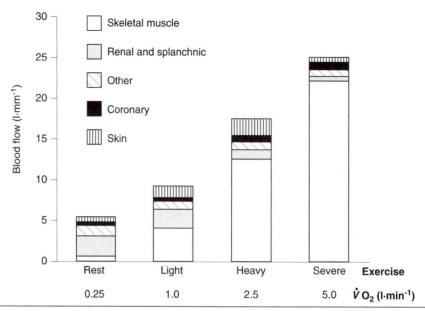

Fig. 2. Bar graph illustrating a redistribution of cardiac output in different levels of dynamic exercise using different amounts of oxygen (oxygen uptake $\dot{V}O_2$)
The changes occurring in different vascular beds suggest a repatterning of sympathetic activity as well as local metabolic effects.

muscle, this would provide only 210 ml of oxygen if the blood was completely desaturated on passing through the muscle. Thus an increase in cardiac output is essential even to do gentle walking. Equally important is the redistribution of blood flow; this may be suitably illustrated by the example of maximal exercise, wherein cardiac output may increase six-fold, e.g. from 5 to 30 litres per min, and enable an overall increase in oxygen uptake of 20 times the resting value. Since this increase in oxygen uptake is mainly occurring in the active muscles, a larger proportion of cardiac output is distributed to these muscles. The alternative would be for the muscles to take the same proportion of a much greater cardiac output. Using the above example, without the blood flow switching to active muscle, cardiac output would have to increase by 20 times, i.e. up to 100 litres per min, to provide the same increase of oxygen uptake: a quite impossible task. The way in which the heart and systemic vascular system adapt to meet this challenge is dependent on the intensity and also the mode of exercise.

Most of our daily activities are composed of two sorts of muscle activity. One is isometric exercise, in which muscles contract without much change in length and there is no joint or axial skeletal movement. Such exercise is performed in lifting, carrying and pushing activities and, therefore, is probably the dominant form of daily exercise encountered in many vocational tasks. By conventional definition, no external work is performed during isometric exercise and the metabolic cost measured in oxygen consumption ($\dot{V}O_2$) is usually modest. However, the high intramuscular tension, owing to contracting muscle fibres, compresses blood vessels, reduces muscle blood flow (Fig. 3) and produces a unique 'pressor' reflex, or increase in arterial blood pressure, which differs substantially from that seen during dynamic exercise performed at an equivalent $\dot{V}O_2$ (Fig. 3) [1,2].

In dynamic exercise, muscles contract and shorten rhythmically and there is movement of joints. Between contractions there is a marked dilatation of muscle blood vessels due to local factors (see Chapter 7); this has profound consequences on vascular resistance (Fig. 3) and on the distribution of blood flow in the systemic circulation (Fig. 2).

The cardiovascular response to each of these modes of exercise is shown for comparison in Fig. 4. A sustained leg extension, at 30%

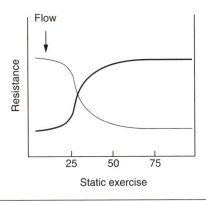
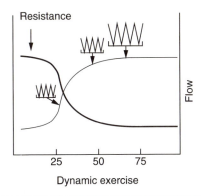

Fig. 3. Schematic illustration of the mean flow (thin line) and mean resistance (thick line) changes occurring in skeletal muscle during static (left) and dynamic (right) exercise at various levels as a percentage of maximum (horizontal axis)

During dynamic exercise the fluctuations in flow, due to rhythmic contractions, as well as the mean flow are indicated by the three expanded portions of the trace.

maximum voluntary contraction gives rise to the response shown in Fig. 4(a). In this example, the increase in $\dot{V}O_2$ is modest (since there is a relatively small muscle mass involved). This is supplied to the muscles by a small increase in cardiac output brought about mainly by an increase in heart rate, which is crucial in this form of exercise since stroke volume often decreases. The mean arterial blood pressure rises quite markedly. The increase in blood pressure is the result of a modest increase in cardiac output and sometimes of an increase in total peripheral resistance, which may increase because the metabolic vasodilatation in the active muscles is over-ridden by the effect of mechanical compression produced by sustained muscle contraction (Fig. 3). In addition, sympathetically induced vasoconstriction occurs in non-active muscle and other vascular beds. As a consequence, diastolic as well as systolic pressure is increased quite markedly (Fig. 4a).

Rhythmic dynamic exercise of both legs on a bicycle ergometer produces a quite different pattern of cardiovascular response, as illustrated in Fig. 4(b). In this example, the active muscles have a relatively high demand for oxygen. This is provided by a large increase in cardiac output to which an increase in heart rate and stroke volume contribute. The increase in stroke volume, due to an increase in activity in sympathetic nerves to the myocardium, is maintained by increased right atrial filling (venous return) brought about by the pumping activity of the leg muscles and the dramatic fall

	Rest	(a) Isometric (30% MVC)	(b) Dynamic (82% $\dot{V}O_2$ max.)
$\dot{Q}$ (l·min^{-1})	5.7±3	6.8±7	21.9±1
HR (beats·min^{-1})	70±7	110±6	164±4
SV (ml)	85±7	62±5	131±5
MAP (mmHg)	94±3	118±6	124±4
TPR (dyn·s·cm^{-5})	1352±3	1466±131	461±56

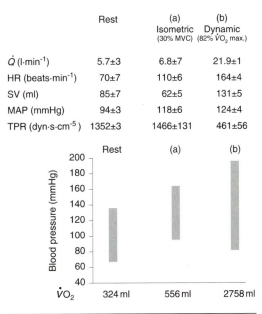

Fig. 4. Measurements of cardiac output ($\dot{Q}$), heart rate (HR), stroke volume (SV), mean arterial pressure (MAP) and total peripheral resistance (TPR) for a group of eight subjects who performed the exercises below

(a) Isometric (static) exercise at 30% of maximum voluntary contraction (MVC) was performed by extending one leg for 3 min. (b) Dynamic exercise involved the use of two legs. The graph shows the mean systolic and diastolic blood pressures (bars), measured for the two types of exercise with a catheter in a brachial artery. Adapted from [2].

in systemic vascular resistance, mostly due to the active muscle vasodilatation.

In this form of exercise there is usually a large increase in systolic pressure and a fall or no change in diastolic pressure. The mean arterial blood pressure is, therefore, only modestly increased. The potential for greater increases in pressure is dampened by a large decrease in systemic vascular resistance (Figs. 3 and 4). Blood is diverted away from the splanchnic and renal vascular beds and non-active muscle by sympathetically mediated vasoconstriction. At first, skin blood flow is reduced but it then increases in parallel with the increasing heat load; during prolonged heavy exercise this may well result in a decrease in the proportion of cardiac output distributed to the active muscles. Under these conditions, skin blood flow can rise from 0.5 to 2 litres or more. However, in very severe exercise, skin blood flow is again reduced and a greater proportion of cardiac output goes to the active muscles (Fig. 2). Thus, the pattern of changes in the cardiovascular system in both modes of exercise depends on autonomic nerve activity interacting with local haemodynamic events.

▶ When muscles contract rhythmically for long periods, the increase in oxygen consumption is provided by an increase in cardiac output and a redistribution of blood flow, which favours the active muscles. Both factors are crucial in optimizing performance.
▶ The changes in the cardiovascular system are dependent on a repatterning of sympathetic nerve activity and withdrawal of cardiac vagal tone.
▶ Exercise can involve two sorts of muscle activity: isometric (or static) contractions and dynamic (or rhythmic) contractions.
▶ In general, isometric contractions result in an increase in total peripheral resistance and an increase in heart rate so that there is often a large increase in mean arterial blood pressure.
▶ Dynamic exercise is accompanied by a decrease in total peripheral resistance, and an increase in stroke volume and heart rate, so that there is a large increase in cardiac output but mean arterial pressure only rises modestly.

Regulation of the cardiovascular response to exercise

Despite the differences in the cardiovascular adaptations that occur with the two types of exercise (shown in Fig. 4), the cardiac output in response to both isometric (<50% maximum voluntary contraction) and isotonic exercise is strongly coupled to the absolute VO_2 [2] (Fig. 5). This close association between muscle metabolism or oxygen usage and cardiac output strongly suggests an active feed-back control mechanism which is similar for both types of exercise. To ensure the right degree of autonomic activity and cardiorespiratory matching, the central nervous system must have information about the degree of muscle activity. There are five ways by which this information transfer could be achieved (Fig. 6). Four of the ways are reflexly induced and are dependent on afferent

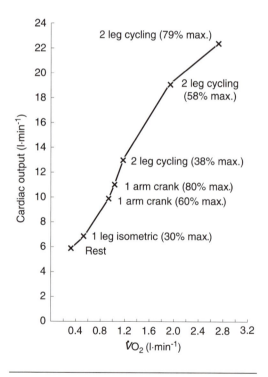

Fig. 5. **Relationship between cardiac output and oxygen consumption (VO_2) during various modes of exercise**
The increase of cardiac output with oxygen consumption is linear regardless of the type of exercise performed. Adapted from [1].

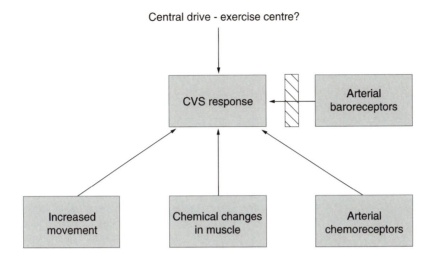

Central drive - exercise centre?

Fig. 6. Diagram summarizing the various factors influencing the cardiovascular (CVS) response to exercise

The hatched bar across the baroreceptor arrow is to indicate that the efficacy of the reflex may be reduced.

input from either joints, muscles, arterial chemoreceptors or arterial baroreceptors. A fifth way suggests that the cardiorespiratory changes associated with movements are initiated as part of the central motor command from the brain to the skeletal muscles.

Role of joint afferents

Passive movements of the limbs have been shown to elicit an increase in ventilation and this is reduced following joint anaesthesia. However, it is now known that such movements are accompanied by small increases in $\dot{V}O_2$ suggesting that muscle activity accompanies the passive movements. This has thrown into doubt the significance of joint afferent contribution to the cardiorespiratory changes during exercise. However, more recent studies [3] in animals like the cat have established beyond reasonable doubt that limb movement can stimulate joint receptors to produce cardiorespiratory changes. Passive movements of the hindlimbs elicited increases in heart rate and in arterial blood pressure in proportion to the number of joints that moved (Fig. 7). All the changes were abolished or significantly reduced after section of the nerves from the joints. The cardiovascular events were still present when animals were paralysed and artificially respired, indicating that joint receptors might contribute

about 10% of the drive to the cardiovascular and respiratory changes, since these changes were so much smaller when evoked by 'passive' movement than when the muscles were also active. Thus it could be that input from the joints facilitates the exercise responses when the rate and extent of joint movement is sufficiently large.

Role of muscle afferents

The suggestion that the cardiovascular response to muscular exercise in man is dependent on a reflex from the exercising muscle is quite an old one, dating from the late nineteenth century. Since these early observations, several pieces of evidence have strongly favoured the muscle reflex hypothesis.

Most of the evidence has come from studies using isometric muscle contractions because these lend themselves more easily to experimental manipulation than do rhythmic contractions of muscles, and because the conditions of the experiments can be more rigorously controlled. Although the cardiovascular changes are different in the two forms of exercise (see above) the sensory input to the central nervous system that produces them is likely to be the same. In view of the close relationship between muscle metabolism or oxygen consumption and the magnitude of the cardiorespiratory changes, it would seem logical in a well-designed control system that the sensory receptor would be in the muscle itself. In humans, there are two observations in particular that suggest that this is likely to be the case.

The first of these is that both heart rate and blood pressure increase linearly in proportion to the intensity of isometric muscle contraction, and these changes are potentiated when the contractions are elicited during occlusion of the circulation to the muscles. This was first elegantly demonstrated with forearm muscles

contracting at 10%, 20% and 50% of the maximum voluntary contraction [4–6] (Fig. 8). Secondly, several groups of investigators have shown that the increase in these cardiovascular variables is also proportional to the mass of muscle contracting. For example, in a comparison of three static exercise manoeuvres involving increasing muscle mass, hand grip, leg extension and dead lift, heart rate and mean arterial blood pressure increased progressively [4,7,8] in proportion to each activity (Fig. 9).

The reflex mechanism for the cardiovascular response to isometric contractions of limb muscles was firmly established in animal experiments [9,10]. In these experiments, the muscles were made to contract by stimulating the appropriate ventral roots. Sectioning the relevant dorsal roots, i.e. removing the afferent supply from the muscles, or paralysis of the muscles abolished the cardiovascular responses (Fig. 10).

The nature of the muscle receptor

Like the responses to voluntary sustained contraction (recorded in humans), the cardiovascular response to ventral root-stimulated muscle contractions in animals was potentiated by prior occlusion of the blood supply to the muscles [9, 10]. It was also proportional to the tension developed by the contracting muscles as well as to the mass of muscle contracting. These features of the reflex suggest that the pertinent muscle receptors may be responding to both mechanical and chemical stimuli arising in the contracting muscle. The muscle afferent fibre population, connected to spindles and Golgi tendon organs, does not contribute to the reflex. Rather, the relevant receptors may be pressure-sensitive receptors [10–12] with small, myelinated afferent fibres. These are probably responsible for the initial reduction in vagal tone which leads to an increase in heart rate [13]. However, the major afferent drive is probably from unmyelinated afferents excited by some locally produced substance, such as potassium, which is in high concentration in the interstitium during muscle contraction (see Chapter 7). These afferents certainly respond to sustained muscle contraction and are powerfully excited by intra-arterial injection of K^+ [12].

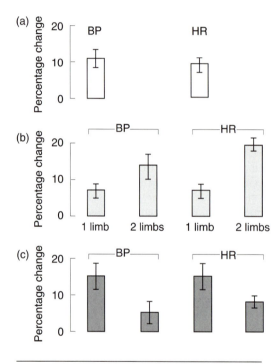

Fig. 7. The cardiovascular effect of rhythmic passive movements of the limbs

Histograms show changes in mean blood pressure (BP) and heart rate (HR) induced by cycling movements of the hindlimbs of decerebrate, unanaesthetized cats. Open columns in (a) show the results of eight experiments in which one limb was moved passively (120 rev./min for 3 min). Light shaded columns in (b) show the effect of moving first one limb (left-hand column) and then reciprocal movement of both hindlimbs (right-hand column) in three experiments. Darker shaded columns in (c) compare the changes resulting from movement of one partially denervated limb before (left-hand column) and after (right-hand column) section of the articular nerves of the knee joint in four experiments. Reproduced with permission from [3].

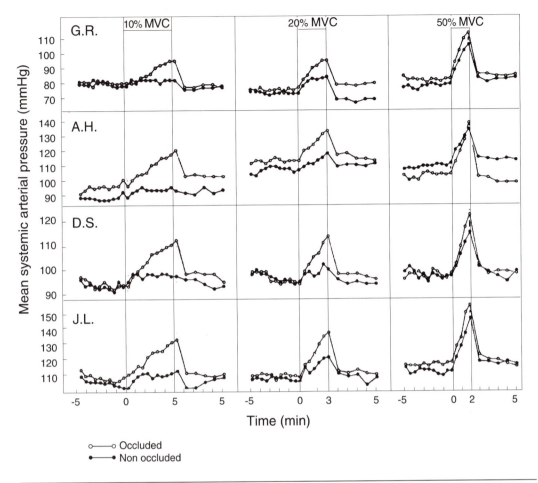

Fig. 8. Evidence for a muscle reflex
Changes in systemic arterial pressure during 10%, 20% and 50% of maximum voluntary contraction (MVC) of arm muscles (hand grip) in four humans during free circulation (closed circles) and during vascular occlusion (open circles) of the exercising arm. Occlusion of the blood supply was affected only for the period of isometric contraction, by inflating a cuff around the upper arm to 240 mmHg. Reproduced with permission from Staunton, H.P., Taylor, S.H. and Donald, K.W. (1964) Clin. Sci. 27, 283–291.

▶ Animal studies have clearly shown that afferent fibres activated by movements of the joints or contractions of muscles can elicit cardiovascular changes similar to those accompanying exercise.
▶ The magnitude of the cardiovascular events is linearly related to the number of moving joints and to the tension developed in muscle contraction, as well as to the mass of muscle contracting.

▶ The afferent fibres involved are the smaller diameter fibres, the myelinated Group III and the unmyelinated Group IV connected to mechanoreceptors and metaboreceptors.

Central nervous drive

There is, therefore, no doubt that muscle afferents can elicit cardiorespiratory changes of the sort accompanying exercise. But how much of

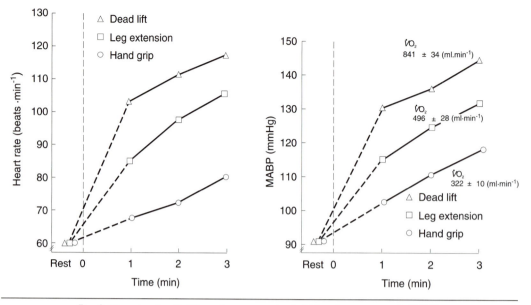

Fig. 9 **Heart rate (left) and mean arterial blood pressure (MABP) (right) responses to static contractions (30% of maximum voluntary contraction) of 3 min duration with increasing muscle mass**
$\dot{V}O_2$ *is the oxygen consumption measured during the third minute of each manoeuvre. Reproduced with permission from [5].*

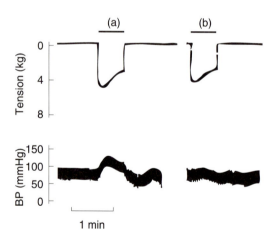

Fig. 10. **Reflex nature of the pressor response to static contraction**

Anaesthetized cat showing records of tension (top) and arterial blood pressure (BP) (bottom) developed by triceps surae during tetanic contraction of right hindlimb muscles elicited by stimulating peripheral cut ends of ventral roots L6–S1, before (a) and after (b) section of dorsal root L6–S1. Reproduced from [9] with permission.

the response in human subjects is due to this afferent feed-back? This question is important because there is an old idea that the cardiorespiratory changes associated with movements are initiated as part of the motor command from the brain to the muscles. Studies in animals have shown that cardiorespiratory changes similar to those that occur during exercise can be elicited by stimulating regions of the brain [14,15], such as the subthalamic area (fields of Forel), from which co-ordinated walking or running movements are also evoked [16]. This has fuelled the idea that the cardiovascular responses accompanying sustained muscle contractions in humans are partly, if not entirely, evoked by a central nervous drive that is commonly referred to as central command. Inherent in this argument is the fact that cardiovascular changes should be present even when command signals are given to muscles that are unable to respond. Consistent with this it was shown that blood pressure and heart rate still increased in subjects attempting to make hand grips with an arm paralysed with succinylcholine [17]. In addition, the magnitude of the evoked cardiovascular response is thought to be related to the degree of perceived effort. An elegant series of experiments has been designed to test this. In one experiment, individuals were asked to make voluntary contractions of a given force. Tendons were then vibrated, activating muscle spindles and thus reflexly assisting or inhibiting the voluntary isometric contractions [18] (Fig. 11). The cardiovascular response evoked by reflexly assisted contractions (Fig. 11b) was less than that evoked by unassisted contractions. In contrast, the cardiovascular response was greater when the muscle contraction was reflexly inhibited (Fig. 11a). In another series of experiments, maximal muscle strength was reduced by partial curarization [18]. This resulted in a greater cardiovascular response for the same absolute force (Fig. 12). These experiments seemingly support the idea that the cardiorespiratory response is proportional to the degree of effort; however, there are a number of criticisms that can be directed at this type of experimental approach. In many of the studies, the effects possibly produced by respiratory changes were not discounted (see Chapter 2), neither were any of the procedures sufficiently rigorous to rule out the possibility of alternative muscle groups assisting the contractions. It is surprising that none of the studies chose to measure oxygen uptake ($\dot{V}O_2$) to ensure that this was the same under all experimental condi-

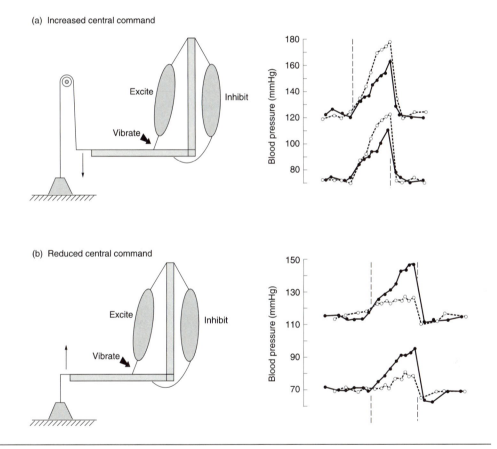

Fig. 11. **The influence of central command**
The systolic and diastolic blood pressure changes in humans during isometric contractions. (a) Isometric contractions of triceps with (open circles) and without (closed circles) vibration of the biceps tendon to reflexly inhibit the triceps, and hence increase the effort to reach the same degree of tension as in control contraction (increased central command). (b) Isometric contraction of biceps. The responses to a normal contraction are shown by the filled circles and continuous lines; the responses when vibration was applied to biceps tendon to reflexly assist contraction, and hence reduce effort required to reach same tension as control (reduced central command), are shown by open circles and dashed lines. Reproduced with permission from [18].

tions. As described earlier, the cardiovascular changes induced by contracting muscles are linearly proportional to the $\dot{V}O_2$.

Some support for the above criticism comes from experiments attempting to increase central command by reducing the efficacy of motor fibres to muscle in human volunteers by spinal anaesthesia, so decreasing muscle strength [19] (Fig. 13). This is a procedure whereby a local anaesthetic solution, such as lidocaine, is injected epidurally to block sensory fibres of dorsal roots. The anaesthetic will also block motor fibres in ventral roots and will affect several spinal segments. Thus this proce-

dure will produce muscle weakness as well as a fairly widespread reduction in afferent feedback from muscles other than those used as part of the study. In such experiments (see Fig. 13b), the cardiovascular and respiratory changes elicited by submaximal contractions of the same absolute force as in the controls were no different to the controls (Fig. 13b) despite the greater effort (central command) required to reach the test tension. Hence a more extensive afferent 'denervation' led to the conclusion that the changes were reflexly induced.

The importance of muscle afferents has been further emphasized in studies taking

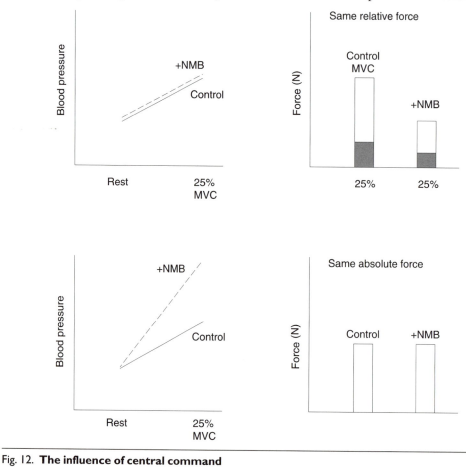

Fig. 12. **The influence of central command**

Diagram to illustrate an experiment in which human subjects performed static contractions of the quadriceps femoris of one leg with the same relative and absolute force (in Newtons, N) before (solid lines) and after (dashed lines) partial neuromuscular blockade (+ NMB), which reduced strength to about 50% of the maximal voluntary contraction (MVC) indicated by height of columns. During the contractions with the same absolute force (lower graphs and open columns; i.e. more effort required), the magnitude of the blood pressure response was greater during NMB than during control contractions. During the contractions involving the same relative force (filled part of each column; i.e. same degree of effort), the magnitude of the blood pressure response was almost the same as control. Adapted from [24] with permission.

another ingenious approach in which the cardiovascular changes were examined in the absence of central command [20]. This has been achieved in two ways (see Fig. 14). First, by studying the changes at the end of a voluntary muscle contraction, with and without occlusion of the circulation to the muscle group. Secondly, by comparing the effects with those at the end of involuntary contraction (induced by electrical stimulation of muscle), with or without occlusion of the circulation to the muscle group. Comparable blood pressure rises occurred during voluntary and involuntary contraction, and during circulatory arrest (Fig. 14b). The drop in arterial blood

pressure at the end of contraction was significantly reduced by circulatory arrest (Fig. 14b). Therefore, it appears that trapping metabolites in the muscle by occluding its blood supply maintains an elevated blood pressure after both voluntary and involuntary contraction: strong evidence in support of the muscle reflex hypothesis. A slight twist to the story has been the observation that vascular occlusion did not maintain the heart rate response to muscle contraction (Fig. 15a). Furthermore, unlike the pressor response, the heart rate response is unaffected when the afferent input from dynamically active muscles is prevented by epidural anaesthesia [7] (Fig. 15b). However,

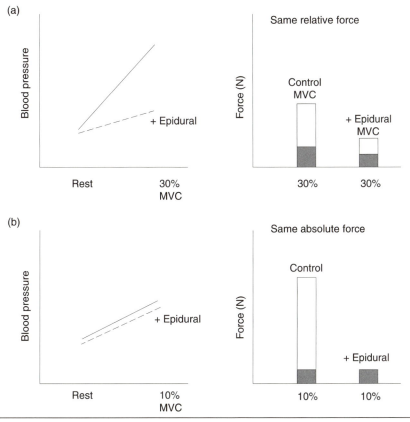

Fig. 13. Diagram to illustrate an experiment in which humans performed static contractions of knee extensors in one leg with the same relative and absolute force (Newtons, N) before (solid lines) and during (dashed lines) epidural anaesthesia which reduced strength to around 60% of the maximal voluntary contraction (MVC)

(a) During the contractions with the same relative force (filled part of the columns; same intended effort but less force of contraction), the increases in blood pressure were less during epidural anaesthesia than during control contractions. (b) During contractions of same absolute force (lower graphs) there was no significant difference in the magnitude of the blood pressure responses between control contractions (10% of absolute force; filled part of column) and those of equivalent force performed during epidural anaesthesia. Adapted from [19] with permission.

neither of these findings necessarily shows that central command is essential for the cardiac changes. Clearly, central command could not have been operating in the involuntary contractions, where the pattern of the cardiac and blood pressure change was essentially similar to that during voluntary contractions. However, the reason for the rapid decrease in heart rate at the end of both voluntary and involuntary contractions (Fig. 15a), even when the circulation to the muscles was occluded, is unclear. It could indicate that a metabolic substance passing from the active muscles into the circulation is

also important. The rebound increase in heart rate on releasing the occlusion, which is significant for involuntary contractions, supports this possibility.

In some circumstances, cardiovascular changes anticipate muscular activity, which is a clear indication that central command plays a part in the autonomic responses to exercise. The most convincing arguments for this have come from recent experiments. Mental effort has been shown to increase heart rate and blood pressure in proportion to imagined load in circumstances where there is no detectable

(a)

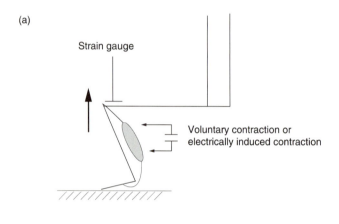

(b)

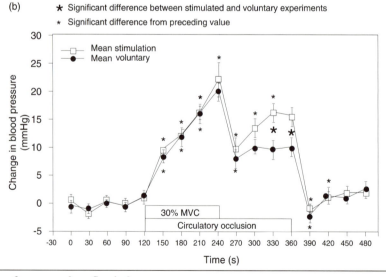

Fig. 14. Evidence for a muscle reflex in humans
(a) Voluntary or electrically induced isometric contractions of triceps surae at 30% of maximum tension (MVC) measured via a strain gauge. (b) The graph shows the similarity between the peak diastolic pressure induced by both methods (open symbols, electrically induced; closed symbols, voluntary contractions) and the sustained elevation of blood pressure at the end of contraction when the circulation to and from the leg was occluded. Adapted from [20] with permission.

increase in metabolism [21] or in subjects with total neuromuscular blockade [22].

Therefore, it seems likely that both peripheral mechanisms and central command contribute to the cardiovascular events during volitional exercise.

The role of central command

A rather elegant test of the relative roles of the central and peripheral inputs was designed by Rowell and co-workers [23,24]. These authors postulated that the important function of a muscle 'chemoreflex' is to raise arterial blood pressure (or, more precisely, to raise cardiac output which might lead to an increase in blood pressure and hence perfusion pressure) whenever blood flow falls below some critical level, causing metabolism in the muscle to become anaerobic. In a series of experiments on conscious dogs, the hypothesis was examined by graded partial occlusion of the blood supply to the hindlimb (terminal aorta), so as to reduce

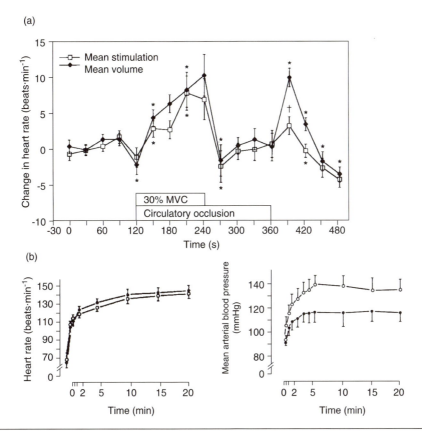

(a)

(b)

Fig. 15. Evidence that the heart rate response to muscle contraction involves different mechanisms to the blood pressure response

(a) Isometric contractions. Heart rate change in response to electrically induced (open symbols) and voluntary (closed symbols) isometric contractions of the triceps surae at 30% maximum tension (MVC). Data given as mean ± S.E.M. (n = 9). Significant difference from preceding value * and † indicates significant difference between stimulation and voluntary experiments. Reproduced with permission from [20]. (b) Dynamic exercise of legs. Heart rate (left) and mean arterial blood pressure (right) responses to 20 min sub-maximum exercise (57% maximum oxygen uptake) in six healthy subjects with (closed symbols) and without (open symbols) epidural anaesthesia. Values given are mean ± S.E.M. Resting values given for epidural anaesthesia were obtained 30 ± 6 min after administration of epidural anaesthesia and immediately before onset of exercise. Reproduced with permission from Fernandez, A., Galbo, H., Kjaer, M., Mitchell, J.H., Secher, N.H. and Thomas, S.N. (1990) J. Physiol. **420**, 281–293.

blood flow in a stepwise fashion during different levels of exercise on a treadmill (Fig. 16). It was demonstrated that, consistent with the hypothesis, at moderate and more severe levels of exercise (Fig. 16a), as flow was decreased by graded occlusion, systemic arterial blood pressure rose steeply and linearly to restore blood flow. However, during mild exercise (Fig. 16b), the pressor response was only mildly facilitated despite a large initial drop in hindlimb blood flow, and the subsequent increase in blood flow was small. Thus the operating point of the response is on a flat slope (see Fig. 16b). A further degree of occlusion which produced a stepwise change in flow [below a threshold (*T*), see Fig. 16b] again caused a steep rise in blood pres-

sure, similar to the facilitation seen during moderate exercise (see Fig. 16a), which restored blood flow. This suggests that there are two components in the regulatory mechanisms causing the pressor response of muscular exercise. One is a pressure-raising response elicited as part of the motor command, enabling increases of muscle blood flow during mild exercise when the margin for blood flow error is large (operating point shown in Fig. 16b). The other control is masked during higher levels of exercise when the muscle chemoreflex becomes tonically active because of a persistent metabolic error signal, i.e. the margin between metabolic needs and blood flow is small (operating point is on a steep slope, see Fig. 16a).

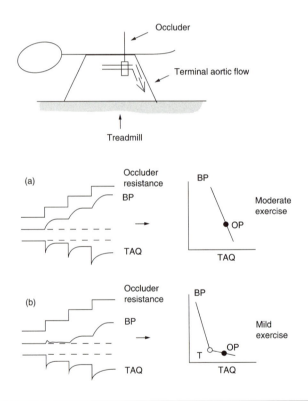

Fig. 16. Schematic diagram of a functional test of the muscle chemoreflex hypothesis

Top diagram illustrates the experiment with a dog on a treadmill. (a) Graded increments in resistance across an occluder on the terminal aorta during a moderate level of exercise will reflexly elicit graded increments in systemic arterial pressure (BP) that will partially restore terminal aortic flow (TAQ) to the exercising muscles. The operating point (OP) is on the steep slope relating BP and TAQ, i.e. if flow is reduced there is a significant rise in BP to try to compensate by increasing perfusion pressure. This sug- *gests that at this level of exercise there is a tonically active muscle reflex. (b) A similar series of graded increments in resistance during a lower level of exercise (mild). At first, flow is allowed to decrease more because there is little increase in BP; this is shown by the rather flat slope for the operating point. BP will not rise until TAQ falls below some critical value, a threshold T, at which the muscle reflex becomes active. Reproduced with permission from [24].*

▶ The cardiovascular changes accompanying exercise are dependent not only on afferent feed-back from muscle and joints but also on a feed-forward mechanism provided by central motor command signals, which as well as initiating movements also activate vasomotor regions of the brain.

▶ It appears likely that motor command plays a significant part during mild exercise, but other mechanisms are more important during moderate and severe exercise.

Role of arterial chemoreceptors

There have been many attempts to explain the matching of cardiorespiratory changes with the intensity of exercise in terms of feed-back from the peripheral arterial chemoreceptors. The chemoreceptors sense the oxygen and carbon dioxide tension and the H^+ concentration of the arterial blood. Unless exercise becomes very severe, these factors hardly change. In the late 1970s, a novel idea was proposed which took account of the well-known rate sensitivity of the carotid body chemoreceptors. It was pointed out that although mean partial pressure of arterial CO_2 ($PaCO_2$) does not change during exercise, it does fluctuate throughout the respiratory cycle, increasing during expiration and decreasing during inspiration. During exercise, increases in frequency and depth of respiration would result in an increase in the rate and magnitude of the change in $PaCO_2$, even though mean $PaCO_2$ would remain unchanged. Unfortunately, there is no evidence for such a mechanism causing the cardiovascular changes; it has even proved difficult to show clearly that CO_2 oscillations are a key factor in eliciting the respiratory events during exercise. However, they could play a part in helping to maintain the respiratory drive later in exercise. Whatever the mechanism, the idea that $PaCO_2$ oscillations alone have an important role has gone out of favour, after the discovery that changes in arterial K^+ concentration could be a powerful additional stimulus to chemoreceptors [25–28].

The venous drainage from working muscles contains increasing amounts of K^+ lost from muscle cells, and the amount is in proportion to the intensity of contraction and to the number of active muscles. This K^+ reaches the arterial blood and, in man, the arterial concentration can double during severe exercise and shows a positive correlation with ventilation. The levels of K^+ reached are similar to those that significantly increase ventilation in the anaesthetized cat by exciting the carotid body chemoreceptors [29]. In addition, experiments in anaesthetized cats [28] show that there is a linear positive correlation between arterial K^+ concentration and respiratory minute volume which is abolished by sectioning the carotid sinus afferent nerves. Hence the respiratory changes during exercise could be partly dependent on changes in arterial K^+ concentrations. It is unclear whether a contribution is also made to the cardiovascular changes. Usually in experimental animals circulatory responses have a much higher threshold for carotid body stimulation than do the respiratory events. Whether the enhancement of carotid chemoreceptor discharge to changes in $PaCO_2$, PaO_2 or pH is large enough to reach a level of activity normally required to elicit significant cardiovascular changes is largely unresolved. Nonetheless, a contribution from the chemoreceptor afferents — subliminally exciting pools of vasomotor neurones and thus potentiating the effects of other inputs — is a likely possibility. In addition, the chemoreceptors may have indirect effects on cardiac and vasomotor neurones via the respiratory system. Thus an increase in central respiratory drive has been shown in the cat to result in a central inhibition of cardiac vagal neurones (Fig. 17), which would increase heart rate [30] (see Chapter 2). It still remains to be shown that such a mechanism operates in humans.

▶ The activity of arterial chemoreceptors may be enhanced during exercise by raised arterial K^+ originating from contracting muscles. This will contribute to the increase in ventilation during exercise by increasing central respiratory drive.

▶ Animal studies indicate that central inspiratory neurones inhibit cardiac vagal neurones and thus, during exercise, an increase in heart rate would be reinforced by this mechanism.

▶ Vascular changes could also be facilitated by increased excitatory input to vasomotor neurones from the arterial chemoreceptors.

Role of arterial baroreceptors

It has been considered that in dynamic exercise the large increase in muscle vascular conductance leading to a decrease in total peripheral resistance would cause a fall in mean pressure, and would result in an unloading of the arterial baroreceptors. As a consequence, sympathetic activity to the heart and blood vessels would increase. Although this could be a contributing factor early in rhythmic exercise it certainly could not be so in isometric exercise because arterial blood pressure does not decrease (even initially) in isometric exercise. Probably of more significance is a resetting of the baroreceptor reflex in exercise.

Elevation of mean arterial blood pressure and pulse pressure, together with shortened systolic time, provides a powerful stimulus to the arterial baroreceptors and would normally result in resistance vessel dilatation and bradycardia. Such an action is not evident in exercise and has led to the suggestion that the baroceptor reflex is suppressed during exercise. However, several types of experiment have shown that a decrease in heart rate and in blood pressure produced by stimulation of the baroreceptors was of the same order of magnitude at rest as during exercise, suggesting that the reflex is still operating during exercise.

This seeming paradox was resolved by the introduction of a more elegant approach to analysis of the heart-rate changes by Sleight and co-workers in Oxford [31,32]. If the heart rate is expressed as the change in pulse interval (R–R interval) produced by baroreceptor stimulation, and this is compared before and during exercise, then the slope of the line relating the pulse interval (in ms) to the mean or systolic pressure (in mmHg) is an index of the sensitivity of the reflex (Fig. 18a). In terms of excitability of neurones in the cardiac reflex pathway, this analysis is a more appropriate approach, since the relationship between R–R interval and the frequency of cardiac vagal stimulation is linear, whereas the relationship between heart rate and cardiac vagal activity is hyperbolic. In consequence, an increment in the activity of vagal efferents would prolong the R–R interval by a fixed value independent of the initial R–R inter-

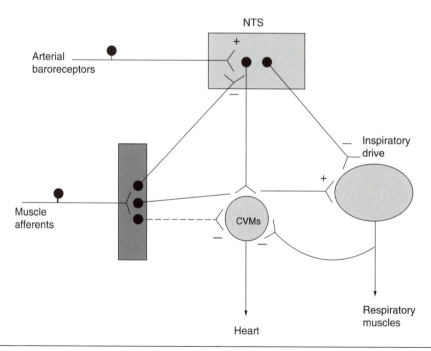

Fig. 17. The influence of a reflex from muscle on the cardiac vagal tone

Diagram illustrating possible ways in which muscle afferents could influence the activity in cardiac vagal neurones (CVM); effect could be either by inhibiting neurones (−) in the primary relay area for the baroreceptors, the nucleus of the tractus solitarius (NTS), or by inhibiting cardiac vagal neurones, or by exciting (+) inspiratory neurones which may then inhibit cardiac vagal neurones. (See also Chapter 2, Fig. 4).

val. Using this approach, stimulation of baroreceptors produces a smaller prolongation of the R–R interval during dynamic and isometric exercise than at rest, and, hence, we can conclude that the sensitivity of the baroreceptor reflex is reduced (Fig. 18a and 18b).

This alteration of the baroreceptor reflex is beginning to be understood in terms of events in the cardiac vagal neurone pool in the central nervous system. Studies in both man and animals have shown that a major component of the heart-rate increase early in exercise is a removal of vagal tone. Furthermore, animal studies have clearly shown that ventral root-induced static contraction of muscles to activate muscle afferents can powerfully reduce the efficacy of the arterial baroreceptor influence on vagal tone (Fig. 18b). Three ways by which this might occur are recognized. First, muscle afferent activity could directly reduce the activity in cardiac vagal nerve fibres and hence result in a reduction in the R–R interval (Fig. 17). Secondly, the muscle afferent input could mod-

ulate the influence of the baroreceptor input at the level of the primary relay area in the nucleus tractus solitarius [10]. Thirdly, animal studies have shown that an increased central inspiratory neurone activity (similar to that accompanying exercise) exerts a powerful inhibition on cardiac vagal neurones. This has not so far been unequivocally demonstrated in humans.

> Increases in arterial blood pressure and in heart rate are not so easily suppressed by the arterial baroreceptors during exercise as they are at rest.
> There is a decrease in the sensitivity of the baroreflex control of heart rate during exercise.
> Animal studies have shown that activation of small afferent fibres from muscle can block the baroreceptor reflex.
> These effects will lead to an increase in heart rate and in vasomotor activity.

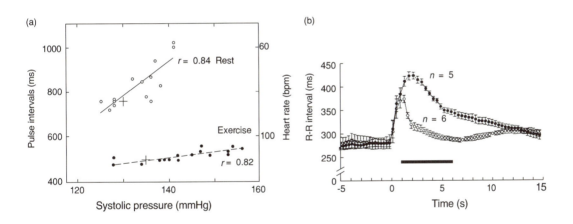

Fig. 18. Contribution of the baroreceptor reflex to the exercise response

(a) Resetting of the baroreceptor–cardiac pulse interval relationship. Points represent pulse intervals resulting from increasing arterial blood pressure by different amounts with infusion of phenylephrine, a peripheral α-adrenergic agonist. Open circles in a resting subject, closed circles in a subject exercising on a bicycle ergometer. During exercise, a drug-induced increase in systolic pressure produces a much smaller increment in the R–R interval than a similar drug-induced change in systolic pressure at rest. Reproduced with permission from [32]. (b) The effect of isometric contraction of hindlimb muscles, elicited by lumbar ventral root stimulation, on pulse interval (mean ± S.E.M.) in a decerebrate cat in which vagal tone was increased by raising carotid sinus pressure to stimulate the arterial baroreceptors. Closed circles indicate the control response to an elevation of carotid sinus pressure alone; open circles show that muscle contraction applied 1 s after the baroreceptor stimulus reduced the R–R change within 1 s, indicating that muscle receptors can block the baroreceptor reflex, and also that the decrease in the R–R interval is probably due to a decrease in cardiac vagal tone. Reproduced with permission from McMahon, S.E. and McWilliam, P.N. (1992) J. Physiol. **447**, 549–562.

Integration of exercise signals

It should now be evident that the response we call the 'exercise reflex', which enables us to perform quite remarkable feats of physical performance, is dependent on an interaction of a number of regulatory mechanisms (Fig. 19). To refer to these as redundant mechanisms misrepresents their true significance. Without an increase in cardiac output and a redistribution of blood flow to the active muscles we would do little more than walk: survival would be impossible. It is, therefore, imperative that the control system has a number of supportive mechanisms to match supply and demand. Each mechanism has a part to play in enabling the efficient functioning of the skeletal muscles which are the key tissues involved in exercise.

The issue which has been much debated is the part played by 'central command' relative to that by peripheral mechanisms. Clearly, the initiation of exercise is a 'voluntary' response and motor command is essential. The evidence that signals for motor command also set up cardiovascular and respiratory systems to initially match the energy needs of exercising muscle is substantial and has been greatly reinforced by two recent, well-controlled studies [21,22]. In addition, the idea of feed-back from the working muscles (metaboreceptor concept) control-

ling their perfusion is attractive and also has a sound experimental basis. Thus a mismatch between muscle blood flow and metabolism will alter the concentration of metabolites in the muscle. This change is detected by chemosensitive nerves in the muscle, and their altered firing pattern 'informs' the central nervous system about the adequacy of muscle perfusion. In as much as the increase in cardiac output goes to working muscle, feed-back from a 'metabolic sensor' in the muscle could provide a precise way of matching blood flow to metabolism. Furthermore, the metabolites (CO_2, lactate and K^+) also pass from the working muscle into the circulation to stimulate the peripheral arterial chemoreceptors. Ideally, then, any metabolic error signal would be continuously corrected by the autonomic nervous system. Joint and muscle afferents, in addition to the direct effects on cardiovascular neurones, may directly influence activity of respiratory neurones which will then reduce cardiac vagal neurone activity and possibly increase medullary vasomotor neurone activity. Although more evidence for these interactions is required, they do serve to illustrate the complexity of the operational system.

Together these mechanisms, both central and peripheral, enable a more precise matching of muscle blood flow to the work being performed.

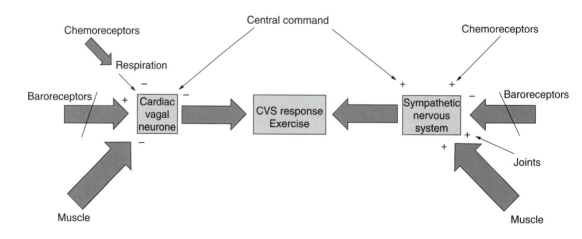

Fig. 19. **Diagram summarizing the way in which various factors interact in the cardiovascular response to exercise**
(+) Indicates excitation; (-) indicates inhibition.

References

References [4,5,23–26,31] are review articles.

1. Bezucha, G.R., Lenser, M.C. and Hanson, P.G. (1982) Comparisons of haemodynamic responses to static and dynamic exercise. J. Appl. Physiol. **53**, 1584–1592

2. Hanson, P.G. and Nagle, F. (1987) Isometric exercise: cardiovascular responses in normal and cardiac populations. Cardiol. Clin. **5**, 157–170

3. Barron, W. and Coote, J.H. (1973) The contribution of articular receptors to cardiovascular reflexes elicited by passive limb movement. J. Physiol. **235**, 423–436

4. Mitchell, J.H., Blonquist, C.G., Lind, A.R., Saltin, B. and Shepherd, J.T. (1981) Static (isometric) exercise: cardiovascular responses and neural control mechanisms. Circ. Res. **48**, Suppl. I, 1–188

5. Mitchell, J.H. and Schmidt, R.F. (1983) Cardiovascular reflex control by afferent fibres from skeletal muscle receptors. In Handbook of Physiology, Vol. 3, Section 2 (Shepherd, J.T. and Aboud, F.M., eds.), pp. 623–658, Am. Physiol. Soc., Washington

6. Lind, A.R., Taylor, S.H., Humphrey, S.P.W., Kennelly, B.M. and Donald, K.W. (1964) The circulatory effects of sustained voluntary muscle contraction. Clin. Sci. **27**, 229–244

7. McCloskey, D.I. and Streatfeld, K.A. (1975) Muscular reflex stimuli to the cardiovascular system during isometric contractions of muscle groups of different mass. J. Physiol. **250**, 431–441

8. Seals, D.R., Hanson, P.G. and Washburn, R.A. (1983) Increased cardiovascular response to static contraction of larger muscle groups. J. Appl. Physiol. **544**, 434–437

9. Coote, J.H., Hilton, S.M. & Perez-Gonzalez, J.F. (1971) The reflex nature of the pressor response to muscular exercise. J. Physiol. **215**, 789–804

10. McCloskey, D.I. and Mitchell, J.H. (1972) Reflex cardiovascular and respiratory responses originating in exercising muscle. J. Physiol. **224**, 173–186

11. Kaufman, M.P., Longhurst, J.C. and Rybicki, K.J. (1983) Effects of static muscular contraction on impulse activity of groups III and IV afferents in cats. J. Appl. Physiol. **55**, 105–112

12. Kniffki, K.D., Mense, S. and Schmidt, R.F. (1978) Responses of group IV afferent units from skeletal muscle to stretch, contraction and chemical stimulation. Exp. Brain Res. **31**, 511–522

13. Hollander, A.P. and Bouman, L.N. (1975) Cardiac acceleration in man elicited by a muscle-heart reflex. J. Appl. Physiol. **38**, 272–278

14. Eldridge, F.L., Millhorn, D.E., Kiley, J.P. and Waldrop, T.G. (1985) Stimulation by central command of locomotion, respiration and circulation during exercise. Respir. Physiol. **59**, 313–337

15. Smith, O.A., Rushmer, R.F. and Lasher, E.P. (1960) Similarity of cardiovascular responses to exercise and to diencephalic stimulation. Am. J. Physiol. **198**, 1139–1142

16. Marshall, J.M. and Timms, R.J. (1980) Experiments on the role of the subthalamus in the generation of the cardiovascular changes during locomotion in the cat. J. Physiol. **301**, 92–93

17. Secher, N.H. (1985) Heart rate at the onset of static exercise in man with partial neuromuscular blockade. J. Physiol. **368**, 481–490

18. Goodwin, G.M., McCloskey, D.I. and Mitchell, J.H. (1972) Cardiovascular and respiratory responses to changes in central command during isometric exercise at constant muscle tension. J. Physiol. **226**, 173–190

19. Mitchell, J.F., Reeves, D.R., Rogers, H.B. and Secher, N.H. (1989) Epidural anaesthetic and cardiovascular responses to static exercise in man. J. Physiol. **417**, 13–24

20. Bull, R.K., Davies, C.T.M., Lind, A.R. and White, M.J. (1989) The human pressor response during and following voluntary and evoked isometric contraction with occluded local blood supply. J. Physiol. **411**, 63–70

21. Decety, J., Jeanerod, M., Durozard, D. and Baverel, G. (1993) Central activation of autonomic effectors during mental simulation of motor actions in man. J. Physiol. **461**, 549–563

22. Gandevia, S.C., Killian, K., McKenzie, D.K., Crawford, M., Allen, G.M., Gorman, R.B. and Hales, J.P. (1993) Respiratory sensations, cardiovascular control, kinaesthesia and transcranial stimulation during paralysis in humans. J. Physiol. **470**, 85–107

23. Rowell, L.B. (1993) Human Cardiovascular Control. Oxford University Press, Oxford

24. Rowell, L.B. and Sheriff, D.D. (1988) Are muscle 'chemoreflexes' functionally important? News Physiol. Sci. **3**, 250–253

25. Linton, R.A.F. and Band, D.M. (1990) Potassium and breathing. News Physiol. Sci. **5**, 105–107

26. Paterson, D.J. (1992) Potassium and ventilation in exercise. J. Appl. Physiol. **72**, 811–820

27. Linton, R.A.F. and Band, D.M. (1985) The effect of potassium on carotid chemoreceptor activity and ventilation in the cat. Respir. Physiol. **59**, 65–70

28. Linton, R.A.F. and Band, D.M. (1988) The relationship between arterial pH and chemoreceptor firing in anaesthetised cats. Respir. Physiol. **74**, 49–54

29. Burger, R.E., Estavillo, J.A., Kumar, P., Nye, P.C.G. and Paterson, D.J. (1988) Effects of oxygen, carbon dioxide and potassium on the steady-state discharge of cat carotid body chemoreceptors. J. Physiol. **401**, 519–531

30. Lopes, O.U. and Palmer, J.F. (1976) Proposed respiratory 'gating' mechanism for cardiac slowing. Nature (London) **264**, 454–456

31. Eckberg, D.L. and Sleight, P. (1992) Human baroreflex in health and disease. Monogr. Physiol. Soc. vol. 43, Clarendon Press, Oxford

32. Bristow, J.D., Brown, E.B., Cunningham, D.J.C., Howson, M.G., Petersen, E.S., Pickering, T.G. and Sleight, P. (1971) Effect of bicycling on the baroreflex regulation of the pulse interval. Circ. Res. **28**, 582–592

7

Metabolic control of blood flow with reference to heart, skeletal muscle and brain

Margaret D. Brown
Department of Physiology, The Medical School, University of Birmingham, Birmingham, B15 2TT, U.K.
Present address: School of Sport and Exercise Sciences, University of Birmingham, Birmingham B15 2TT, U.K.

Introduction

The main aim of the circulation is to ensure a proper milieu for cells by supplying oxygen and substrates for tissue respiration and by removing waste metabolites. It follows that if blood supply is less than that required to meet functional demands of an organ/tissue, metabolism will be compromised by lack of oxygen and accumulation of metabolites, leading to cell dysfunction. Alterations in metabolic demand at the organ level are met by changes in the level of perfusion; for example, the proportion of cardiac output received by the skeletal muscle mass increases 3–4-fold upon change from rest to exercise (see Chapter 6). The idea of metabolic control of blood flow involves a feed-back system, in which blood vessels controlling organ perfusion are responsive to some metabolic error signal, presumably a substance or substances produced in the tissue as a result of mismatch between metabolic supply and demand. Metabolic control of blood flow relates not only to the way in which increases in metabolic need are met by appropriate changes in blood flow (functional hyperaemia), but also to situations in which oxygen/substrate supply is inadequate, e.g. by impairment of perfusion. As such, it ensures matching between supply and demand and is, therefore, evident not only in situations of functional hyperaemia but also in hypoperfusion where supply is compromised (reactive hyperaemia). It can also contribute to autoregulation, the maintenance of organ blood flow in the face of changes in perfusion pressure; for example, if perfusion pressure is increased, vasodilator metabolites would be 'washed out', leading to vasoconstriction.

Metabolic control is only one of the regulatory mechanisms which determine blood flow and, therefore, interacts with neural, myogenic, hormonal and physical influences upon vascular smooth muscle. However, it plays an important role in determining the capacity of three important organs — heart, brain and skeletal muscle — to function under conditions of widely varying metabolic activity, and the study of these provides us with the opportunity to investigate what it is that actually couples blood flow to metabolism.

Relationship between blood flow and metabolism in heart, brain and skeletal muscle

The ratio between the proportion of total body oxygen consumption required by individual organs and the proportion of cardiac output that each receives demonstrates that the closest matching between metabolic requirements for oxygen and blood flow occurs in heart, brain and skeletal muscle. In other organs, e.g. kidney and skin, flow is in excess of metabolic requirements and subserves other functions, such as filtration and heat dissipation. Resting levels of blood flow are higher in heart (approx. 70 ml/min per 100 g in humans) and brain (50–60 ml/min per 100 g) than in skeletal muscle (2–15 ml/min per 100 g), in proportion to resting oxygen consumption (8 and 3 ml/min per 100 g for heart and brain, respectively, and <1 ml/min per 100 g for skeletal muscle).

In the heart, the main determinants of oxygen consumption are contractility, heart rate and ventricular wall tension, and, since resting oxygen extraction is already high (75%), it is more-or-less totally dependent upon increases in flow (4–5-fold) to meet oxygen demand during activity, showing a good correlation between blood flow and oxygen consumption [1]. The large mass of skeletal muscle (about 40% of body weight) also requires profound circulatory adjustments during muscle activity to accommodate up to 25-fold increases in blood flow. Resting oxygen extraction is lower than in the heart (around 25–30%) and increased oxygen consumption during muscle activity can, therefore, be met by increased oxygen extraction (up to 80–90%), in addition to increased flow. Although individual skeletal muscles display considerable heterogeneity in the metabolic profile of their constituent fibres and their vascular supply, the correlation between oxygen consumption and blood flow broadly holds [2]. In both heart and skeletal muscle, blood flow is subject to intermittent impedance by mechanical compressive forces, which occlude it particularly in the subendocardium during systole and in skeletal muscle during tetanic contractions (see Chapter 6).

Total brain blood flow is relatively constant, and it was not until the advent of methods for flow and metabolism measurement, with sufficient spatial resolution to detect regional heterogeneity, that the tight metabolic regulation of perfusion at the local level became apparent. Such methods include Kety–Schmidt inhalation of diffusible indicators, [^{14}C]-antipyrine, radiolabelled microspheres, positron emission tomography and computer-assisted reconstruction, [^{14}C]-2 deoxyglucose and quantitative autoradiography for glucose utilization as an index of metabolism. With these techniques it could be shown that, while there is little change in oxygen extraction over a range of blood flow, there is a close correlation between local metabolic rate and cerebral blood flow in both experimental animals and humans. Localized increases in blood flow during different types of cerebral activity are accompanied by flow decreases in other areas [3].

Possible factors involved in metabolic regulation of blood flow

The basic idea of metabolic regulation of blood flow is that there are vasoactive products released from active cells which influence the smooth muscle cells of blood vessels. Possible substances linking metabolism and blood flow (oxygen, K$^+$, carbon dioxide, lactate, pH, adenosine, inorganic phosphate and osmolarity) have been described in several reviews of the subject (for example, see [4]). The search for one single factor linking metabolism to blood flow is clearly inappropriate because of the variability in degree to which metabolic control operates under different conditions, such as hypoxia, reactive hyperaemia and functional hyperaemia, and also because this presupposes that factors pertaining when the supply side is compromised (e.g. hypoxia, reduced perfusion) would necessarily be the same as when the demand side is increased (functional hyperaemia). It is also possible that different factors are involved in the initiation of vasodilatation from those which maintain it during prolonged metabolic activity.

The site of action of any of these metabolic products should ultimately be on smooth muscle cells of the arteriolar resistance vessels (Fig. 1) where there are several possible modes of action. There could be a local effect either on the vessel outer wall, or a local indirect effect by

---

Table I Criteria for identification of possible couplers between cell metabolism and blood-flow

- There should be an adequate source of the substance occurring naturally in the tissue.
- The substance should have access to vascular smooth muscle.
- The concentration of the substance in interstitial fluid should be sufficient to produce and maintain dilatation.
- The substance should be shown to be a potent vasodilator *in vitro* and *in vivo*.
- Antagonists/inhibitors or potentiators of the substance should be shown to have the appropriate effects, i.e. blocking or enhancing, upon its exogenous and endogenous effects.

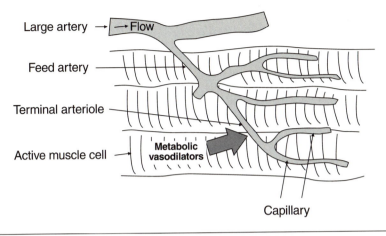

Capillary

Fig. 1. Site of action of metabolic vasodilator substances
It is generally assumed that the ultimate site of action of metabolic vasodilators must be on the smooth muscle of the terminal resistance arterioles which regulate capillary flow.

interaction with neural elements, or a substance or substances released at a distance from the resistance vessels could act on them via the blood-stream or some other signalling means. The mechanism of vasodilator action is likely to be by influencing Ca^{2+} entry into smooth muscle cells via voltage-operated or receptor-operated channels — possibly involving ATP-sensitive K^+ channels [5].

A list of criteria by which possible mediators of metabolic vasodilatation could be identified was originally proposed by Mellander and Johansson [6] and has since been refined [7] (Table 1). Although these criteria still remain as the basis for establishing a metabolic vasodilator coupler, there are some important considerations. The first two criteria are self-evident, but it should be noted that the second implies the presence of the substance in the interstitial fluid, not necessarily in venous effluent. The third criterion is more difficult to substantiate for technical reasons. In many cases it has been assumed that measuring the concentration of a substance in venous effluent is indicative of its presence and concentration in the interstitium, but this may not be the case if there is cellular uptake of the substance by tissue and/or endothelial mechanisms (e.g. for adenosine in heart), or variations in capillary permeability to released substances which may restrict venous efflux. The fourth criterion can be established

by several experimental means. The substance should produce vasodilatation when applied to isolated tissue or vessel preparations where pharmacological characterization of responses can be made; alternatively, observations of its direct effects on resistance vessels can be made *in vivo* in preparations such as the cranial window for pial vessels, trans- or epi-illuminated skeletal muscle preparations and even on epicardial surface vessels in the heart. If infused intra-arterially or intravenously, the substance should produce a comparable degree of vasodilatation with a similar time-course to that occurring naturally. However, such experiments may not accurately represent the effects of the substance in its interstitial compartment and should be interpreted in the light of factors which could affect its access to smooth muscle. The use of antagonists/inhibitors or potentiators of the substance in the intact organ can demonstrate its involvement but may be difficult to interpret if abolition of the effects of one substance expose the action of another.

Evidence for the role of putative metabolic vasodilator substances

Oxygen
Blood vessels show some intrinsic sensitivity to oxygen. For example, when arterial partial

pressure of oxygen (PO_2) is reduced below about 40 mmHg, vascular resistance decreases in skeletal muscle, brain and heart. Responsiveness to hypoxia is observed in isolated vessels from the heart and skeletal muscles, and pial vessels dilate rapidly to either low PO_2 or superfusion with cerebrospinal fluid (CSF) at low PO_2. Superfusion of pial vessels with a fluorocarbon solution at high arterial PO_2 reduces the dilatation to low arterial PO_2, suggesting that oxygen lack can play a role in regulation of cerebral vessel tone. In addition, diameter changes in response to changes in superfusate PO_2 have also been observed in resistance arterioles in skeletal muscle prepared for intravital microscopy.

Oxygen lack has been discounted as a metabolic vasodilator on the basis that arterial blood vessel walls are exposed to high arterial PO_2 levels on their luminal surface. However, it could be the oxygen gradient that exists across the vessel wall between blood and tissue levels which is important (Fig. 2). Two critical ques-

tions have to be answered to establish a role for oxygen in metabolic vasodilatation. The first is whether the tissue PO_2 levels to which smooth muscle cells would be exposed abluminally accurately reflect metabolic energy state and, secondly, if so, whether a lack of oxygen influences vessel tone by direct action on vascular smooth muscle or indirectly via release of vasodilator metabolites. When oxygen supply is compromised by arterial hypoxia, tissue PO_2 measured directly by microelectrodes decreases in all three tissues — heart, skeletal muscle and brain — but a reduction in coronary perfusion pressure may only increase heterogeneity of tissue PO_2 rather than reduce it overall. On the other hand, increases in metabolic activity have varied effects on tissue O_2 — it has been shown to decrease in skeletal muscle during and after contractions, not to change in myocardium at different work levels achieved by moderate lowering and raising of heart rate, and to rise in brain when neuronal activity is increased by stimulation or seizures. Thus it is not clear that during increased metabolic activity, lack of oxygen at the tissue level occurs to a sufficient degree in heart or brain to initiate functional hyperaemia. The main evidence against a role for oxygen lack as a direct initiator of metabolic vasodilation in skeletal muscle comes from observations that, during contractions, arteriolar diameters increased before any decrease in tissue PO_2 was observed [8].

The time-course of changes in venous PO_2 does not always correlate with that of vascular resistance in skeletal muscle undergoing either brief tetanic or prolonged contractions. This may be because a discrepancy exists between venous and tissue oxygen levels, especially at low arterial PO_2. A similar discrepancy is found in the heart, between the time-course of changes in vasodilatation and venous PO_2. For example, reactive hyperaemia is proportional to, but in excess of, the initial oxygen debt, persisting even after coronary sinus oxygen levels have approached arterial levels. Although coronary sinus PO_2 has been taken to reflect tissue levels in the heart in some studies, others have observed a delay in venous PO_2 changes relative to cardiac tissue PO_2. Further, coronary blood flow does not increase in response to a reduction in oxygen content of arterial blood if flow is maintained by high perfusion pressure and coronary sinus oxygen levels are above resting. This suggests that oxygen lack is not

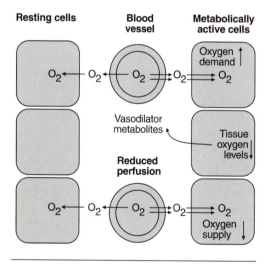

Fig. 2. Role of oxygen as a putative metabolic vasodilator

Smooth muscle cells in the blood vessels could be sensitive to tissue levels of PO_2. These would be altered by supply/demand mismatch. Metabolically active cells can increase their demand for oxygen and hence oxygen flux (double arrows). If this is not met by increased supply, for example, if perfusion is reduced, it would lead to reduced tissue levels of oxygen and subsequent release of vasodilator metabolites (curved arrow), or altered PO_2 gradients between tissue and blood (large versus small O_2 symbols).

the primary cause of vasodilatation, and is effective only under conditions of low flow. On the other hand, it has been reported that anoxic perfusion can produce a similar peak increase in flow as coronary occlusion [9].

▶ Although there is evidence of an intrinsic sensitivity of blood vessels to oxygen, it is unlikely that during increased metabolic activity tissue oxygen levels fall sufficiently and/or quickly enough to account for vasodilatation.

▶ Lack of oxygen does not appear to be directly involved in blood flow regulation unless flow is restricted. Under these circumstances, it is more likely that release of one or more vasodilator metabolites is involved.

▶ Hypoxia may modulate responsiveness of vessels to other metabolites.

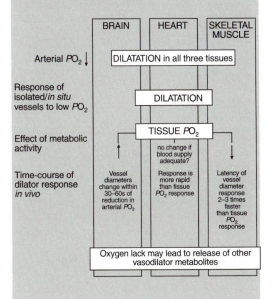

Carbon dioxide, pH and lactate

Interstitial accumulation of carbon dioxide and lactate, and a fall in pH are consequences of increased cellular metabolic activity (Fig. 3) and they have been considered as potential candidates for metabolic coupling to blood flow.

Hypercapnia results in a decrease in vascular resistance, most notably in the cerebral circulation. In comparison, skeletal muscle blood flow seems to be relatively insensitive to changes in arterial PCO_2. Perfusion of hindlimb muscle with blood at high PCO_2 has minimal effects on blood flow, and carbon dioxide release from actively contracting muscle is not considered sufficient to account for functional hyperaemia. Similarly, the effects of changes in PCO_2 on coronary circulation appear to be variable and inconclusive. In general, experiments in heart and skeletal muscle have not discriminated between direct effects of carbon dioxide on vessels, or indirect effects mediated by the associated reduction in interstitial pH, which could influence vascular smooth muscle activity by altering intracellular Ca^{2+} handling. However, elimination of tissue acidosis in the ischaemic myocardium did not alter arteriolar dilatation, indicating that acidosis does not play a major role in coronary reactive hyperaemia [10]. In active skeletal muscle, the change in hydrogen ion concentration [H⁺] is considered too small to account for changes in vascular resistance during exercise (see Chapter 6) and there is a lack of correlation between the time-course of changes in venous or interstitial pH and muscle blood flow. Although significant increases in venous blood lactate occur in skeletal muscle during exercise, lactate infusion does not produce dilatation. The most often cited evidence against a role for either lactate, pH or

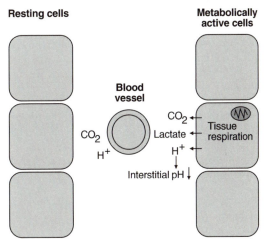

Fig. 3. Carbon dioxide, pH and lactate as putative metabolic vasodilators

Mitochondrial respiration augments production of carbon dioxide, and anaerobic production of ATP in the cytoplasm results in formation of lactate acid and carbon dioxide, both of which diffuse out of the cell and cause an increase in [H⁺] of extracellular fluid, decreasing its pH.

carbon dioxide in muscle metabolic vasodilatation is from patients with McArdle's syndrome, who have an inborn deficiency of phosphorylase enzyme and, consequently, no muscle glycolysis. During muscle contractions there are no changes in venous lactate, pH or PCO_2, yet functional hyperaemia still occurs [11]. It is possible, however, that low pH in active muscle normally plays a facilitatory role by augmenting vasodilatation in response to, for example, low PO_2 or by facilitating enzymes which produce vasodilator polypeptides. Moreover, in heavy exercise, when oxygen supply to tissues is compromised, H^+ ions derived from lactate may be important for promoting oxygen diffusion to mitochondria by a combination of effects, via the Bohr shift and local microvascular dilation. Substances associated with acidosis in active muscles are also important as chemical stimuli to afferent nerve fibres involved in reflex cardiovascular adjustments to exercise, such as the rise in arterial pressure (see Chapter 6).

In contrast, cerebral vessel tone is profoundly affected by alterations in arterial PCO_2; hypercapnia, as a result of inspiration of 5–7% carbon dioxide, increases blood flow by 50–100% and produces dilatation with rapid onset; pial diameter changes are detectable within 1–2 min of increasing inspired carbon dioxide. Several findings indicate that these responses are mediated via changes in extracellular $[H^+]$ as a consequence of carbon dioxide readily crossing the blood–brain barrier. Blood flow is not changed significantly when arterial pH is altered independently of PCO_2, but dilatation does occur if pH is changed by altering bicarbonate ion concentration $([HCO_3^-])$. Also, pial arteries dilate and constrict to acid and alkaline cerebrospinal fluid, respectively, while alterations in $[HCO_3^-]$ or PCO_2 independently of pH have no effect.

To establish a role for extracellular $[H^+]$ in cerebral functional hyperaemia, appropriate changes should be observed during increased metabolic activity. Although pH decreases and cerebral blood flow increases during increased neuronal activity due to electrical stimulation or pharmacologically induced seizures, there appears to be a time lag before the onset of pH changes which would rule out changes in $[H^+]$ as an initiator of metabolic vasodilatation. Hence it is more likely to be important in flow regulation in later stages of neuronal activity.

Changes in extracellular H^+ and lactate concentrations in the brain do not occur to a sufficient degree for these substances to play an important role in control of blood flow during either hypoxia or autoregulation [12].

▶ Neither carbon dioxide, pH nor lactate plays a significant role in metabolic vasodilatation in heart and skeletal muscle.
▶ In the cerebral circulation, carbon dioxide is a potent regulator of vascular tone via its effect on $[H^+]$, but the time-course of changes makes it unlikely to act as an initiator of functional hyperaemia.

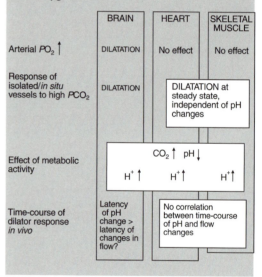

Potassium

Potassium ions are released from excitable cells with the passage of the action potential and, as such, represent a good candidate for the initiation of functional hyperaemia. On a longer term basis, K^+ could be released via K_{ATP} channels and in association with anaerobic glycolysis in muscle (Fig. 4). In vitro, coronary vessels and isolated heart preparations show dose-dependent dilatation over the range of K^+ concentration $[K^+]$ found in tissue (4–16 mM) with a transient response. In the heart *in vivo*, the rate of release of K^+ alters with changes in rate and force of contraction. However, tissue levels of K^+ have not been found to correlate with coronary vasodilatation, and intracoronary infusions of K^+ which markedly elevate plasma concentration increase coronary blood flow only modestly. While this evidence does not

Resting cells　　　　**Metabolically active cells**

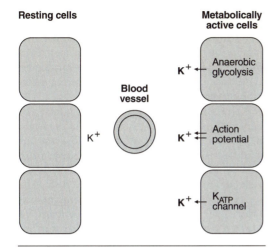

Fig. 4. Role of potassium as a putative metabolic vasodilator

[K⁺] in the extracellular space is increased by depolarization of the muscle/neuron cell membrane, and anaerobic glycolysis leads to K⁺ efflux via ATP-modulated K⁺ channels (K_{ATP}).

strongly implicate K⁺ in the maintenance of coronary functional hyperaemia, in one study, the changes in interstitial [K⁺] calculated during step increases in heart rate preceded vasodilatation and could account for a considerable portion of the initial increases in blood flow [13].

In skeletal muscle, venous K⁺ efflux is reported to show a good correlation with contraction frequency, and with decreases in vascular resistance in both short- (minutes) and long-duration (one hour) contractions [14]. Direct measurements of interstitial [K⁺] in contracting muscle show K⁺ levels to be 30–50% greater than in venous plasma, possibly due to the significant uptake into muscle cells via a β_2-receptor-regulated Na⁺/K⁺-ATPase pump, and this uptake could contribute to the finding that close arterial application of K⁺ in skeletal muscle decreases vascular resistance by only 25% of that seen during exercise. The increase in interstitial [K⁺] with single twitches was previously considered too small in relation to the significant increases in blood flow. However, more recently, small but significant increases in venous [K⁺] were seen after single weak contractions in human muscle of a magnitude (0.9 mM) and time-course sufficient to implicate K⁺ in the initiation and regulation of functional hyperaemia [15]. On the other hand, topical application of K⁺ at concentrations equalling those found in contracting muscle

(9–10 mM) produced maximal arteriolar dilatation in hamster cremaster and rat spinotrapezius muscle preparations, yet the latency of response was found to be too long (15 s) for K⁺ to be the initiator of functional hyperaemia [16]. It should be noted that these muscles are more planar (thin and flat) than, and may respond differently from, those bulkier, locomotory skeletal muscles in which force generation is more significant. In addition to a possible role as vasodilator, K⁺ released from contracting muscle may also be important for stimulating peripheral chemoreceptors, and thus increasing ventilation during exercise (see Chapter 6).

Cerebral vessels dilate when K⁺ is applied in the range of 0–10 mM and stimulation of the brain by electrical or chemical means leads to an increase in extracellular [K⁺] of sufficient magnitude (from 3 to 7 mM), while blood flow increases 4–5-fold. The increase is early and rapid but is transient, possibly due to the potent uptake mechanisms in glial cells for K⁺, and K⁺ has therefore been considered to be an initiator of functional hyperaemia but not to have persistent effects [17].

▶ K⁺ could initiate functional hyperaemia in brain and, possibly, in heart or skeletal muscle.
▶ K⁺ is only likely to be involved in maintenance of dilatation in skeletal muscle.
▶ K⁺ efflux during hypoxia has been demonstrated in both brain and hindlimb muscles, indicating a role in vasodilation when oxygen delivery is impaired.

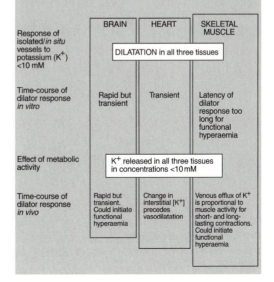

	BRAIN	HEART	SKELETAL MUSCLE
Response of isolated/*in situ* vessels to potassium (K⁺) <10 mM	DILATATION in all three tissues		
Time-course of dilator response *in vitro*	Rapid but transient	Transient	Latency of dilator response too long for functional hyperaemia
Effect of metabolic activity	K⁺ released in all three tissues in concentrations <10 mM		
Time-course of dilator response *in vivo*	Rapid but transient. Could initiate functional hyperaemia	Change in interstitial [K⁺] precedes vasodilatation	Venous efflux of K⁺ is proportional to muscle activity for short- and long-lasting contractions. Could initiate functional hyperaemia

Inorganic phosphate

Inorganic phosphate (P_i) is released from metabolically active cells as a product of ATP breakdown (Fig. 5) and was proposed as a mediator of functional hyperaemia in skeletal muscle on the basis of a good correlation between maximal vascular conductance and P_i efflux from active muscle after short periods of either twitch or tetanic contractions, although the correlation was not sustained during longer periods [14]. Injections or infusions of P_i in its acid (NaH_2PO_4), but not in its neutral form, could mimic functional hyperaemia with a rapid onset in fast muscles. Topical application of P_i dilated skeletal muscle resistance vessels with a short latency [16], but other workers failed to find increases in venous P_i concentration after very brief (5 s) muscular contractions [15] and infusions of P_i into human limbs raised venous concentration without effect on blood flow.

Osmolarity

The osmolarity of the extracellular fluid surrounding metabolically active tissue is increased by the production of osmotically active ions and metabolites. In brain, although topical application of hypertonic and hypotonic solutions dilates and constricts pial arteries, respectively, correlations between brain activity, extracellular osmolarity and cerebral

blood flow have not been clearly defined. No increase in coronary sinus osmolarity was observed on stellate ganglion stimulation, and hyperosmolarity produced only transient relaxation of coronary artery strips.

The strongest support for a role of increased osmolarity in functional hyperaemia in skeletal muscle came from observations of increases in venous blood osmolarity, from 4 to 40 mosm/l, which were graded with the frequency of muscle stimulation [18]. The hyperaemia could be mimicked by infusion of hypertonic solution; however, the latency of responses of arterioles in muscle preparations to topical application of hypertonic solutions is too great (10–20 s) and the magnitude too small (<50% maximal dilatation) to implicate osmolarity as an initiator of functional hyperaemia [16]. Neither would it contribute to maintenance of hyperaemia in view of the lack of correlation between changes in vascular conductance and plasma osmolarity during prolonged muscle contractions [14].

> ▶ P_i has only been investigated in skeletal muscle in relation to functional hyperaemia.
> ▶ In view of the action of P_i in muscle only in the acid form, it may be that it functions in concert with other factors, including pH.
> ▶ P_i has not been considered in metabolic control of blood flow in either heart or brain, although it has been shown to increase to 170% of control values during a brief coronary occlusion.
> ▶ Changes in extracellular osmolarity seem unlikely to be involved in the initiation of functional hyperaemia, and their role in vasodilatation when oxygen supply is restricted is not known.

Adenosine

Adenosine has been considered as a strong candidate for metabolic vasodilator coupling in heart, brain and skeletal muscle since increased release of adenine nucleotides in association with increased blood flow was shown in hypoxic hearts [19]. Adenosine is a powerful vasodilator, formed mainly by dephosphorylation of AMP by 5′-nucleotidase located in the cell membrane. It diffuses rapidly into the interstitial space where it may undergo uptake by cells (both myocytes and endothelial cells in

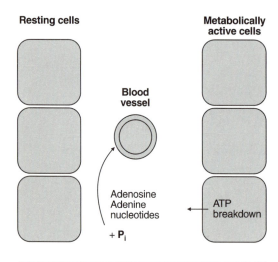

Resting cells

Metabolically active cells

Blood vessel

Adenosine
Adenine
nucleotides

ATP breakdown

+ P_i

Fig. 5. Role of inorganic phosphate as a putative metabolic vasodilator

This is liberated on ATP breakdown, and increases extracellular [P_i].

the heart) and be rephosphorylated and salvaged, or it may be degraded by adenosine deaminase via inosine to hypoxanthine and vaso-inactive metabolites (Fig. 6).

Adenosine release from the heart is detectable in pericardial perfusate in response to exercise, catecholamine stimulation and other interventions which elevate myocardial oxygen consumption. It is also released when oxygen supply is limited by lowering perfusion pressure or coronary artery occlusion. On intracoronary infusion and *in vitro*, adenosine and its analogues are potent vasodilators and there is good correlation between myocardial oxygen consumption, release of adenosine and coronary blood flow both *in vivo* and *in vitro* [19].

Antagonists of adenosine action, such as adenosine deaminase, or theophylline and 8-phenyltheophylline, which block adenosine receptors, have been widely used to verify the role of adenosine in metabolic blood flow regulation. They do not change resting coronary blood flow but partially attenuate vasodilatation during increased myocardial activity, hypoxia and reactive hyperaemia. Several studies using adenosine deaminase have failed to demonstrate an essential role for adenosine in the metabolic component of coronary autoregulation.

Despite the fact that the effects of adenosine antagonists on resting cerebral flow are inconsistent, it has been suggested that there is substantial basal release of adenosine in the brain because dipyridamole, which potentiates adenosine action by blocking its cellular uptake, increases resting flow [20]. Adenosine is released from the brain by electrical stimulation and seizures, and during hypoxia, ischaemia and hypercapnia. Further, adenosine and its analogues relax cerebral vessels on topical application and *in vitro* and may increase cerebral blood flow on intra-arterial infusion. As in the heart, adenosine antagonists reduce but do not abolish functional hyperaemia, but the involvement of adenosine in cerebral metabolic vasodilation is established during oxygen supply/demand mismatch — hypoxia /ischaemia, hypercapnia, severe hypotension and hypoglycaemia — when increases in flow are attenuated by antagonists and potentiated by dipyridamole. It is, however, unlikely to be involved in autoregulation unless oxygenation is inadequate.

Adenosine is released into venous plasma from active skeletal muscles, but mainly after prolonged periods of contraction and particularly if perfusion is limited, so leading to inadequate oxygenation. There is no correlation between venous concentration of adenosine and vascular conductance in hindlimb muscle under conditions of free flow [21]. On the other hand, adenosine is a potent dilator of resistance vessels and adenosine deaminase attenuates muscle functional hyperaemia by around 40%. However, results with adenosine receptor blockers, such as 8-phenyltheophylline, are less conclusive; this drug reduced hyperaemia in contracting cat muscle by 40% but was without effect in conscious dogs [22]. Furthermore, it reduced skeletal muscle vasodilatation during systemic hypoxia, but did not alter reactive hyperaemia in rat cremaster muscle.

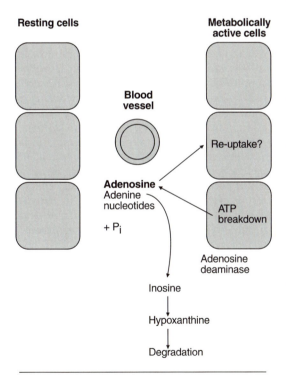

Resting cells

Metabolically active cells

Blood vessel

Re-uptake?

Adenosine
Adenine nucleotides

+ P_i

ATP breakdown

Adenosine deaminase

Inosine

Hypoxanthine

Degradation

Fig. 6. **Role of adenosine as a putative metabolic vasodilator**
ATP breakdown to ADP, AMP and adenosine augments the concentration of adenosine and adenine nucleotides in the extracellular space. The adenosine may be taken up by cells again or undergo degradation by adenosine deaminase.

The main problem with establishment of adenosine as a metabolic vasodilator is the difficulty of obtaining valid estimates of interstitial adenosine levels because of the efficient cellular uptake and degradation mechanism, as demonstrated in cardiac myocytes and coronary endothelial cells [19,23]. For example, arterial infusion of adenosine into the coronary circulation raises its concentration in the interstitium less than in plasma, as these mechanisms effectively compartmentalize adenosine within cells where it would have no access to vasculature. This calls into question both measurements of adenosine release into venous effluent, and attempts at more local extracellular fluid collection by epicardial or cortical superfusate cups. These give more suitable estimates of adenosine interstitial concentration but could cause cellular damage and additional adenosine release [24].

▶ Adenosine is clearly involved in metabolic flow regulation, but the question of whether this is only under conditions of hypoxia needs clarifying.

▶ It is unlikely that adenosine would be an initiator of dilatation but may well be involved in its maintenance.

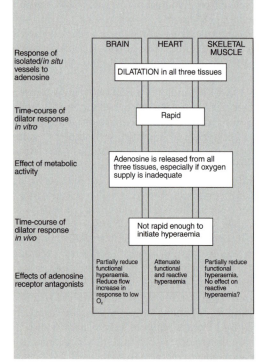

	BRAIN	HEART	SKELETAL MUSCLE
Response of isolated/*in situ* vessels to adenosine	DILATATION in all three tissues		
Time-course of dilator response *in vitro*	Rapid		
Effect of metabolic activity	Adenosine is released from all three tissues, especially if oxygen supply is inadequate		
Time-course of dilator response *in vivo*	Not rapid enough to initiate hyperaemia		
Effects of adenosine receptor antagonists	Partially reduce functional hyperaemia. Reduce flow increase in response to low O_2	Attenuate functional and reactive hyperaemia	Partially reduce functional hyperaemia. No effect on reactive hyperaemia?

In the absence of facilities for on-line analysis of interstitial adenosine concentration for estimation of transient changes, it remains difficult to compare the exact time-course of its release with changes in blood flow during metabolic regulation. Such analysis would also help to elucidate the exact changes in cellular metabolism under which adenosine is released. It has been proposed, from studies of pure cardiac myocyte preparations, that under physiological conditions the levels of adenosine release are very low and that the large amounts of adenosine in the effluent of, for example, isolated hearts are indicative of myocardial damage rather than its role as a physiological regulator of blood flow [25].

Prostaglandins

Prostaglandins (PGs) are compounds derived from fatty acids, such as arachidonic acid, and are produced by almost every type of cell. They are known dilators of cerebral and coronary arteries, and, although they are produced by both brain tissue and cerebral vasculature, their role in metabolic regulation of cerebral flow is still under investigation. While blockade of PG synthesis by indomethacin reduces resting cerebral blood flow by nearly 40%, indicating a basal release, earlier studies showing lack of effect of indomethacin on responses to hypoxia, changes in perfusion pressure and hypercapnia would seem to preclude their involvement in metabolic regulation. However, more recently it has been shown that indomethacin reduces responsiveness of cerebral vessels to carbon dioxide and that products of arachidonic acid metabolism can restore dilatation to hypercapnia.

Administration of different PGs to conscious sheep has been reported to have varying effects (none, constriction or dilation) on hindlimb and coronary vascular beds. In the heart, prostaglandin PGI_2 (prostacyclin) can induce coronary vasodilatation, but, as blockade of its production has little effect on flow, it may be of minor importance in the regulation of perfusion under physiological conditions [26]. Nevertheless, it may modulate coronary vessel responses to sympathetic nerve stimulation and be involved in hypoxic vasodilatation, which is suppressed by indomethacin. In this case, PGs produced by endangered myocardium may counteract vasoconstrictor substances, such as thromboxane.

A review of the evidence for PG involvement in skeletal muscle hyperaemia, either functional or reactive, showed conflicting reports as to their release and whether blockade of their synthesis by indomethacin could alter blood flow [2]. PGs may have a metabolic effect in increasing muscle glucose uptake and utilization. The most likely involvement of PGs in vascular control is their production by endothelial cells in response to increased shear stress on the vessel wall induced by increases in blood flow [27].

▶ The involvement of PGs as primary causative agents of metabolic vasodilatation is not convincing.

▶ PGs are involved as intermediaries producing dilatation in response to endothelially related stimuli, e.g. during flow-induced dilatation, and thus could play a part in the concerted changes within a vascular bed during functional hyperaemia.

The role of endothelium, nitric oxide and vasodilator nerves in metabolic flow regulation

The concept of metabolic vasodilatation embodies the fact that vasoactive metabolites released from active cells act on vascular smooth muscle of resistance vessels to regulate flow through the tissue. However, it is now recognized that endothelial cells lining the blood vessels have a significant role to play in influencing the vascular smooth muscle, and possibly contribute to co-ordination of vasodilatation throughout a vascular bed in a number of different ways. Endothelial cells are responsive to biochemical mediators and physical factors, such as shear stress, received at their luminal surface, and they then mediate vasoactivity in underlying vascular smooth muscle through secondary messengers. This could involve any of a number of substances now known to be produced by endothelium, both dilator, such as endothelium-derived relaxing factor (EDRF), PGs and endothelium-derived hyperpolarizing factor (EDHF), and constrictor, such as endothelin, described in recent reviews (for example, see [28]).

Over recent years, the characterization of EDRF as the endogenous nitrovasodilator, nitric oxide (NO), has opened up a whole new aspect of modulation of vessel tone. NO, formed from L-arginine by the action of the enzyme NO synthase, is released from endothelial cells under basal conditions and in response to various vasoactive stimuli, such as shear stress, platelet-derived factors, hormones and so on. NO is a mediator of endothelium-dependent smooth-muscle relaxation — not necessarily the sole mediator, since prostacylins are also implicated — by activation of soluble guanylate cyclase, leading to production of cyclic GMP. There is an increasing number of studies indicating that NO may be involved in metabolic vasodilatation. Human skeletal muscle expresses NO synthase even more abundantly than brain, and blockade of NO production in both heart and skeletal muscle reduces resting blood flow, indicating a basal release. In skeletal muscle, functional hyperaemia is attenuated by removal of the endothelium or blockade of NO synthesis (by enzyme inhibitors) or its action, and can be increased by addition of the NO precursor L-arginine [29]. However, NO synthesis blockade does not influence reactive hyperaemia or autoregulatory responses. Blockade of NO synthesis also prevents functional hyperaemia in the brain [30]. In the heart, NO production has been shown to be involved in the vasodilator responses to acetylcholine and bradykinin, and to stress and stretch [31], but blockade of NO synthesis does not alter coronary reactive hyperaemia. NO synthase has been demonstrated in the nerves supplying coronary arteries.

There is still much that must be done to define the specific role and sites of involvement of endothelial NO in metabolic vasodilatation, since it is not known whether the involvement of NO is primary in the initiation of metabolic dilatation, or secondary in endothelial-dependent co-ordination mechanisms, in which it is released in response to changes in flow/shear stress. Endothelial cells act as sensors of shear stress and, when blood flow is increased, they respond by production of vasodilator substances, possibly NO or PGs [32], to cause a further dilatation, the so-called 'flow-induced dilatation'. It is also known that the dilator response to metabolites of small arterioles within skeletal muscle can be propagated retrogradely as an 'ascending dilatation' to the larger feed arteries which lie outside the muscle itself, either as a cell-to-cell conducted response or possibly involving shear-stress-related endothelial release of dilator substances [33].

There is considerable heterogeneity in the responses of different segments of a particular vascular bed to vasoactive stimuli. In the heart, for example, metabolic control exerts a dominant effect on the smallest (<20 μm diam.) arterioles, while larger upstream vessels are less responsive to metabolites but more influenced by pressure-induced myogenic mechanisms, and even larger upstream arterial tone is dominated by flow-dependent endothelial mechanisms [34]. The endothelium may, therefore, play an important role in co-ordinating the response of the whole vascular bed to tissue metabolic activity, by aiding communication between these different segments. It has been suggested that during functional hyperaemia, for example, metabolic vasodilators cause preferential dilatation of the smallest arterioles regulating the microvasculature. Upstream arterioles would respond to this reduction in resistance and subsequent increase in flow by 'ascending dilatation' and/or myogenic dilator mechanisms, and the dilatation could spread proximally to larger conduit arteries by endothelial-dependent, 'flow-induced' mechanisms (Fig. 7). This arrangement would permit an integrated response in which flow and perfusion pressure are optimized throughout the whole vascular bed [33].

Although a direct role of endothelium in local metabolic flow regulation remains somewhat speculative at present, it is possible that capillary endothelial cells themselves may be the sensors of metabolic error signals, e.g. local tissue oxygenation, rather than vascular smooth muscle. It has been proposed that coronary capillary endothelial cells could respond to locally produced metabolites and optimize tissue perfusion by signalling spatially and/or temporally integrated responses proximally to their feed arteries [25]. A similar suggestion has been made that microvascular endothelial cells respond to focal increases in metabolism in the regulation of cerebral blood flow [35]. This idea is supported by observations that local application of noradrenaline to a downstream capillary produced constriction of the upstream feed arterioles [36], and that iontophoretic application of acetylcholine to venules produced dilatation of their upstream arterioles in

skeletal muscle, which could be prevented by inhibitors of EDRF [37], indicating a capacity for communication between different segments of the vascular network. The delay between muscle activity and vasodilatation, seen in studies comparing the time-course and magnitude of blood flow changes in human contracting muscle [38], which was explained by diffusion of metabolites to resistance vessels, could then also include time taken for communication between endothelium and arteriole. Whether or not this mechanism could play any role in metabolic regulation of blood flow must await further investigation, and it still leaves open the question of exactly which substances either initiate or sustain the close matching of blood flow to metabolic needs in heart, brain and skeletal muscle.

There is also considerable interest in the possibility that NO may act as a vasodilator neurotransmitter, particularly in cerebral and coronary vessels where nerves to arteries have been shown to contain NO synthase [39]. Indeed, in the cerebral circulation, there is support for the idea that neurogenic rather than metabolic factors are the dominant regulators

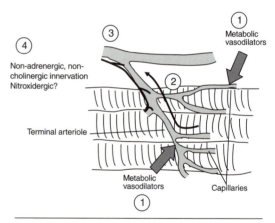

Fig. 7. Possible sequence of events in co-ordination of vasodilatation within the vascular bed during functional hyperaemia
(1) Terminal arterioles and/or capillaries respond to metabolic vasodilators, shown by thick arrows. (2) Signal is conducted retrogradely to feed artery supplying the organ by 'ascending dilatation', shown by thin arrow. (3) Conduit arteries respond via endothelium-mediated, flow-dependent dilatation, thus optimizing flow and perfusion pressure. (4) Initiation of vasodilatation is possibly neurally mediated.

of pial arteries, identified as the prime site of dilatation in functional hyperaemia [40]. Further, Honig [41] supported the role of neurogenic mediation of functional hyperaemia in skeletal muscle after the discovery that intrinsic neurones to the blood vessels remain after a muscle has been extrinsically denervated. Therefore, the possibility re-emerges that it is the innervation to blood vessels themselves that initiates the rapid dilatation in response to increased metabolic activity within an organ. In this context, not only the role of NO as a rapidly synthesized, non-stored, neurally released vasodilator substance, but the proliferation of non-adrenergic, non-cholinergic neurotransmitters, such as Substance P and calcitonin gene-related peptide [42], immediately increases the current list of candidates for initiators of metabolic vasodilatation and expands the possibilities for future research.

Conclusion

> None of the substances which are possible mediators of metabolic vasodilatation satisfies all the criteria necessary to prove its sole involvement in either initiation or maintenance of the hyperaemia, although all the candidates appear to play some role.

> In addition, resistance vessels display differential sensitivities to the possible mediator substances depending on the tissue/organ they supply (e.g. carbon dioxide responsiveness of cerebral versus skeletal muscle or heart vessels), and also on their location within the vascular bed of that particular organ.

> In view of the varied functional requirements and the ways in which these are met by changes in blood flow and/or oxygen extraction in the three organs referred to, some heterogeneity of mechanisms responsible for metabolic vasodilatation is not unexpected.

> It is to be hoped that future research will elucidate more fully the balance of action of the possible mediators within different tissues, and explore the possible contribution of vasodilator neurogenic mechanisms.

M.D.B. was supported by the Wellcome Trust during the preparation of this manuscript.

References

1. Rubio, R. and Berne R.M. (1975) Regulation of coronary blood flow. Prog. Cardiovasc. Dis. 18, 105–122
2. Hudlicka, O. (1985) Regulation of muscle blood flow. Clin. Physiol. 5, 201–229
3. Ingvar, D.H. (1976) Functional landscapes of the dominant hemisphere. Brain Res. 107, 181–197
4. Keatinge, W.R. and Harman, M.C. (1980) Local mechanisms controlling blood vessels. Monogr. Physiol. Soc. Philadelphia 37, 73–77
5. Nelson, M.T., Patlak, J.B., Worley, J.F. and Standen, N.B. (1990) Calcium channels, potassium channels and voltage dependence of arterial smooth muscle tone. Am. J. Physiol. 259, C3–C18
6. Mellander, S. and Johansson, B. (1968) Control of resistance exchange and capacitance functions in the peripheral circulation. Pharmacol. Rev. 20, 117–196
7. Shepherd, J.T. (1983) Circulation to skeletal muscle. In Handbook of Physiology, Vol. 3, Section 2, (Shepherd, J.T. and Abboud, F.M., eds.), pp. 319–370, Am. Physiol. Soc., Bethesda
8. Gorczynski, R.J. and Duling, B.R. (1978) Role of oxygen in arteriolar functional vasodilation in hamster striated muscle. Am. J. Physiol. 235, H505–H515
9. Crystal, G.J. and Downey, H.F. (1987) Perfusion with non-oxygenated Tyrode solution causes maximal coronary vasodilation in canine hearts. Clin. Exp. Pharmacol. Physiol. 14, 851–857
10. Gewirtz, H., Weeks, G., Nathanson, M., Sharaf, B., Fedele, F. and Most, A.S. (1989) Tissue acidosis: role in sustained arteriolar dilatation distal to a coronary stenosis. Circulation 79, 890–898
11. Barcroft, H., Greenwood, B., McArdle, B., McSwiney, R.R., Semple, S.J.G., Whelan, R.F. and Youlten, L.J.F. (1967) The effect of exercise on forearm blood flow and on venous blood pH, PCO2 and lactate in a subject with phosphorylase deficiency in skeletal muscle (McArdle's syndrome). J. Physiol. 189, 44P–46P
12. Busija, D.W. and Heistad, D.D. (1984) Factors involved in the physiological regulation of the cerebral circulation. Rev. Physiol. Biochem. Pharmacol. 101, 161–211
13. Murray, P.A., Belloni, F.L. and Sparks, H.V. (1979) The role of potassium in the metabolic control of coronary vascular resistance of the dog. Circ. Res. 44, 767–780
14. Hudlicka, O. and El-Khelly, F. (1985) Metabolic factors involved in regulation of muscle blood flow. J. Cardiovasc. Pharmacol. 7, S59–S72
15. Kiens, B., Saltin, B., Walloe, L. and Wesche, J. (1989) Temporal relationship between blood flow changes and release of ions and metabolites from muscles upon single weak contractions. Acta Physiol. Scand. 136, 551–559
16. Hilton, S.M., Hudlicka, O. and Marshall, J.M. (1978) Possible mediators of functional hyperaemia in skeletal muscle. J. Physiol. 282, 131–147
17. Kuschinsky, W. (1987) Coupling of function, metabolism and blood flow in the brain. News Physiol. Sci. 2, 217–220
18. Mellander, S., Johansson, B., Gray, S.D., Jonsson, O., Lundvall, J. and Ljung, B. (1967) The effects of hyperosmolarity on intact and isolated vascular smooth muscle: possible role in exercise hyperaemia. Angiologica 4, 310–322
19. Berne, R.M, and Rubio, R. (1979) Coronary circulation. In Handbook of Physiology, Volume I, Section 2, (Berne, R.M., Sperelakis, N. and Geiger, S.R., eds.) pp. 873–952, Am. Physiol. Soc., Bethesda

20. Phillis, J.W. (1989) Adenosine in the control of the cerebral circulation. Cerebrovasc. Brain Metab. Rev. **1**, 26–54

21. Karim, F., Ballard, H.J. and Cotterrell, D. (1988) Changes in adenosine release and blood flow in the contracting dog gracilis muscle. Pfluegers Arch. **412**, 106–112

22. Koch, L.G., Britton, S.L. and Metting, P.J. (1990) Adenosine is not essential for exercise hyperaemia in the hindlimb of conscious dogs. J. Physiol. **429**, 63–76

23. Nees, S. (1989) Coronary flow increases induced by adenosine and adenine nucleotides are mediated by the coronary endothelium: a new principle of the regulation of coronary flow. Eur. Heart. J. **10**, 28–35

24. Olsson, R.A. and Bünger, R. (1987) Metabolic control of coronary blood flow. Prog. Cardiovasc. Dis. **29**, 369–387

25. Nees, S. (1989) The adenosine hypothesis of metabolic regulation of coronary flow in the light of newly recognised properties of the coronary endothelium. Z. Kardiol. **78**, 42–49

26. Bassenge, E. and Heusch, G. (1990) Endothelial and neuro-humoral control of coronary blood flow in health and disease. Rev. Physiol. Biochem. Pharmacol. **116**, 77–170

27. Koller, A. and Kaley, G. (1990) Prostaglandins mediate arteriolar dilatation to increased blood flow velocity in skeletal muscle microcirculation. Circ. Res. **67**, 529–534

28. Vanhoutte, P.M. (1990) Endothelium-derived relaxing and contracting factors. Adv. Nephrol. **19**, 3–16

29. Sagach, V.F., Kindybalyuk, A.M. and Kovalenko, T.N. (1992) Functional hyperemia of skeletal muscle: role of endothelium. J. Cardiovasc. Pharmacol. **20**, S170–S175

30. Goadsby, P.J., Kaube H. and Hoskin, K.L. (1992) Nitric oxide synthesis couples cerebral blood flow and metabolism. Brain Res. **595**, 167–170

31. Ueeda, M., Silvia, S.K. and Olsson, R.A. (1992) Nitric oxide modulates coronary autoregulation in the guinea pig. Circ. Res. **70**, 1296–1303

32. Smiesko, V. and Johnson, P.C. (1993) The arterial lumen is controlled by flow-related shear stress. News Physiol. Sci. **8**, 34–38

33. Segal, S.S. (1992) Communication among endothelial and smooth muscle cells coordinates blood flow control during exercise. News Physiol. Sci. **7**, 152–156

34. Kuo, L., Davis, M.J. and Chilian, W.M. (1992) Endothelial modulation of arteriolar tone. News Physiol. Sci. **7**, 5–9

35. Faraci, F.M. and Heistad, D.D. (1990) Regulation of large cerebral arteries and cerebral microvascular pressure. Circ. Res. **66**, 8–17

36. Dietrich, H.H. (1989) Effect of locally applied epinephrine and norepinephrine on blood flow and diameter in capillaries of rat mesentery. Microvasc. Res. **38**, 125–135

37. Falcone, J.C. and Bohlen, H.G. (1990) EDRF from rat intestine and skeletal muscle venules causes dilatation of arterioles. Am. J. Physiol. **258**, H1515–H1523

38. Wesche, J. (1986) The time course and magnitude of blood flow changes in the human quadriceps muscles following isometric contraction. J. Physiol. **377**, 445–462

39. Snyder, S.H. (1992) Nitric oxide: first in a new class of neurotransmitters. Science **257**, 494–496

40. Baramidze, D., Mchedlishvili, G., Gordeladze, Z. and Levkovitch, Y. (1992) Cerebral microcirculation: heterogeneity of pial arterial network controlling microcirculation of cerebral cortex. Int. J. Microcirc. Clin. Exp. **11**, 143–155

41. Honig, C.R. (1979) Contribution of nerves and metabolites to exercise vasodilatation: a unifying hypothesis. Am. J. Physiol. **236**, H705–H719

42. Owman, C. (1990) Peptidergic vasodilator nerves in the peripheral circulation and in the vascular beds of the heart and brain. Blood Vessels **27**, 73–93

8

Changing perspectives on microvascular fluid exchange

J. Rodney Levick
Department of Physiology, St George's Hospital Medical School, London, SW17 0RE, U.K.

Introduction: importance of fluid turnover

Water and solutes are continuously passing out of the vascular circulation across the walls of capillaries and venules into the interstitial compartment, where they maintain the 'milieu intérieur' of the tissue. The functions of the water input are to maintain tissue hydration; transport large molecules such as immunoglobulins and protein-bound materials (vitamin A, lipids, thyroxine, testosterone, oestradiol, iron and copper) through the tissues; carry antigenic material into the lymphatic system for immunosurveillance; supply water to cells for metabolic use and cell volume regulation; and deliver water for the formation of secretions, such as saliva, pancreatic juice and so on. Water and escaped plasma proteins begin their return journey to the blood-stream by entering fine lymphatic vessels (see Fig. 1) which unite progressively to form afferent lymphatic trunks. When a tissue is in a steady state (constant fluid volume), the rate at which fluid enters the lymphatic system equals the net rate at which it leaves the vascular system. The afferent lymph vessels transport the afferent lymph into lymph nodes, which modify its composition (see later). The fluid draining out of the nodes, called efferent lymph, is carried by efferent lymph trunks to the neck, where the major trunks (principally the thoracic duct) drain directly into veins.

The entire plasma volume (excluding the protein) circulates in the above fashion at least once per day, so the balance between net microvascular filtration rate and lymphatic drainage is a crucial factor governing plasma volume, and hence blood volume (see Chapter 5). Both filtration rate and lymphatic pumping are subject to active control by autonomic, humoral and local mechanisms. Filtration rate can be controlled by regulating arteriolar tone (see Chapter 7), which governs capillary filtration pressure, as explained later. In this way, the rate of loss of fluid from the plasma compartment is brought under the control of the central nervous system and the homoeostatic car-

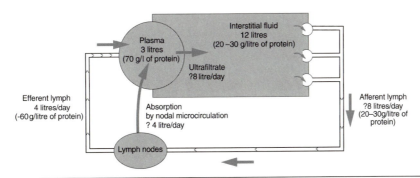

Fig. 1. An overview of the extravascular circulation of fluid in a 65 kg adult
Figures for ultrafiltration rate and afferent lymph flow are rough estimates. Redrawn with permission from [17].

diopulmonary and arterial pressure reflexes (see Chapters 1 and 5).

The filtration rate can be perturbed under a wide variety of conditions, both physiological and pathological, leading to changes in plasma volume. Filtration rate increases in vasodilated exercising muscle (see Chapter 6 and Chapter 7), in heat-dilated skin, in dependent tissues, such as the feet in orthostasis, in a wide variety of oedemas (e.g. cardiac, venous thrombosis and hypoproteinaemic oedemas) and in all inflammatory conditions, including burns and trauma. Conversely, net filtration can be reduced or even reversed to net absorption as part of a protective reflex. The most dramatic example follows severe haemorrhage and produces plasma volume expansion and haemodilution (see Chapter 5) [2].

The basic principles governing the extravascular circulation of fluid were described by Starling in 1896 and confirmed experimentally by Landis in 1927 [3,4]. General textbook accounts of fluid exchange today tend to be brief and somewhat fixated on the classic work of half a century ago, largely ignoring subsequent advances. In keeping with the aims of this volume, an update is presented here. It will emerge that the traditional view, namely that most capillaries are normally filtering fluid from their arterial segments and reabsorbing it in their venous segments, is unlikely to be a true depiction of the steady state in most tissues.

The main theme here is the bulk flow of liquid across the walls of exchange vessels, and the closely related topic of the escape of plasma proteins into the interstitium. The other major role of capillaries, the exchange of solutes such as respiratory gases, nutrients, hormones and so on is dominated by diffusion rather than bulk flow and is not treated here; see [2] for an introductory account and [5,6] for reviews in depth. Before considering exchange at the level of the individual capillary, it is useful to get an overview of fluid turnover rate for the whole body, as described next.

Magnitude of whole-body fluid turnover

The route of passage of extravascular fluid from the capillary to lymph and back is shown schematically in Fig. 1. The estimated magnitude of this extravascular fluid circulation has been increased markedly in recent years. Formerly, the flow of capillary ultrafiltrate through the entire interstitial compartment of an adult man was estimated to be 2–4 litres per day — in itself a very considerable turnover, equivalent to the entire plasma water flowing out of the circulation and back into it each day.

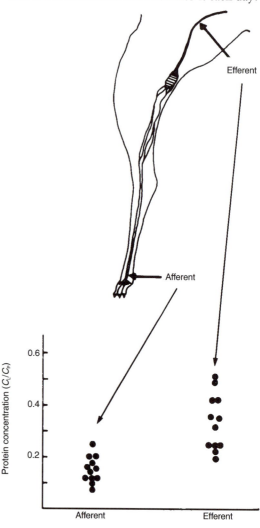

Fig. 2. **Arrangement of lymphatics in hindleg of greyhound (top) and comparison of endogenous plasma protein concentration in afferent and efferent lymphatic vessels (bottom)**

Lymph protein concentration, C_L, is expressed as a fraction of plasma concentration, C_P. Protein concentration approximately doubles during nodal transit, owing to water reabsorption within the node. Reproduced with permission from [7].

Even so, it now appears that this may have been an underestimate, because fluid exchange can take place in lymph nodes.

The thoracic duct carries about 90% of the total body lymph flow, and the traditional estimate of 2–4 litres per day was based on the collection of lymph from accidental fistulae of the thoracic duct in the neck. This lymph, however, is post-nodal or efferent lymph, i.e. lymph that has passed through one or more groups of lymph nodes. This is an important caveat because as lymph passes through lymph nodes its composition and volume can change. Fig. 2 illustrates this; lymph emerging from the dog popliteal node contains a higher concentration of plasma protein than that entering the node. This had actually been known since the work of Kjellmer and Jacobson in 1964, but it had been suggested by Quinn and Shannon in 1977 that the rise in protein concentration was merely due to leakage of protein from capillaries within the node into the lymph. The true, main mechanism was clarified more recently by Adair and Guyton [1] and Knox and Pflug [7],

working independently. They showed that the capillary network within the node absorbs water from the lymph, and, as a result, the lymph emerges with a reduced volume and increased protein concentration. Changes in lymph volume due to nodal transit are shown in Fig. 3, and it will be noted that the degree of 'lymphoconcentration' depends on the vascular pressure within the node. This indicates that intranodal fluid exchange is a passive process that obeys the Starling principle.

The results from popliteal nodes of dog, cat and sheep are clear: up to half of the water in afferent lymph can be absorbed directly into the bloodstream within the node. Consequently, efferent lymph is not, in general, representative of afferent lymph, either in composition or flow. The caveat 'in general' is necessary because in the lung the afferent lymph protein concentration is already nearly 70% of that in plasma, and afferent and efferent lymph have very similar protein levels [8].

It follows that estimates of the extravascular circulation of fluid based on post-nodal

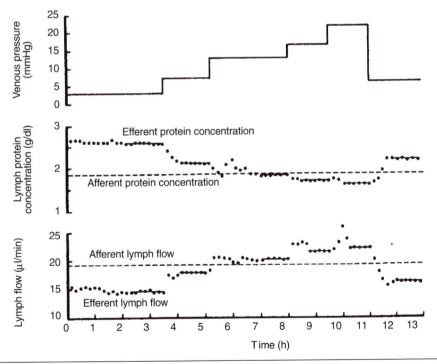

Fig. 3. Proof of fluid exchange within a lymph node

Artificial afferent lymph of fixed protein concentration (dashed lines) was perfused at fixed flow through the dog popliteal node and the efferent flow and protein concentration were measured (points). Volume outflow is less than volume inflow at normal venous pressure, indicating fluid absorption. Raising venous pressure in the node (top trace) reduced the fluid absorption rate. Reproduced with permission from [1].

lymph flow (thoracic duct flow) must be increased. It is not easy to make an exact correction for nodal absorption because the fraction reabsorbed is variable and dependent on local vascular pressure (Fig. 3). Given certain assumptions, however, a revised extravascular circulation was suggested by Renkin (1986) [17]. As Fig. 1 shows, true fluid turnover could be double the former estimate, i.e. 8 litres per day. Of this, 4 litres might be reabsorbed directly into the blood-stream within the lymph nodes, leaving 4 litres to return to the circulation via the major efferent lymph trunks.

Any substantial upward revision of lymph formation rate implies a similar upward revision of net microvascular filtration rate, as shown in Fig. 1. This in turn implies a greater imbalance between filtration and reabsorption at the capillary wall than was formerly believed. This ties in with changes in current concepts of filtration–absorption balance, which have arisen from measurements of the transcapillary driving forces by new techniques and from a better understanding of the dynamic interdependence of transcapillary forces. It is probably no overstatement to declare that the traditional, much-reproduced textbook picture of capillary fluid exchange is out of date and, to a degree, misleading. To explain this challenging statement, the Starling principle must be explored a little more deeply than is usual in textbooks.

> ▶ Up to half the water in pre-nodal lymph can be absorbed by the nodal microcirculation during transit of lymph through a lymph node.
> ▶ Whole-body afferent lymph flow is probably larger than thoracic duct flow (4 litres per day in man). Human net capillary filtration rate could be up to 8 litres per day.

Starling's principle of fluid exchange

The fundamental factors governing microvascular fluid exchange, described by Starling in the Journal of Physiology of 1896 [3,4] are not themselves in doubt. The term 'microvascular' is used to encompass both capillaries and venules because fluid exchange occurs in both kinds of vessel. Starling recognized that the cap-

illary wall functions as a semipermeable membrane, i.e. plasma proteins exert a sustained osmotic pressure across it, while smaller solutes do not. A near balance is struck between the hydraulic pressure of capillary blood, which tends to drive fluid out across the capillary wall, and the colloid osmotic pressure (also called 'oncotic pressure') of the plasma proteins, which tends to suck interstitial fluid into the capillary and oppose blood pressure (Fig. 4). Three important developments of this basic concept have occurred: (i) the introduction of the 'osmotic reflection coefficient'; (ii) the recognition of the importance of extravascular forces (often denied in general textbooks); and, arising from this, (iii) doubt about the concept of upstream filtration–downstream reabsorption along the microvascular axis (the familiar out-and-back-in-again picture). To address these issues, it is helpful to couch the Starling principle in the form of a simple equation (or at least simple looking; appearances can be deceptive, as emerges later).

The Starling principle states that the rate of fluid movement across a small segment of the wall of an exchange vessel (J_v) is proportional, at any point in space and time, to the sum of four pressures: two hydraulic pressures and two

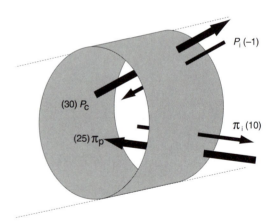

Fig. 4. The Starling principle
Four pressures govern fluid ultrafiltration rate at any given position along the capillary: local capillary pressure, P_c; local interstitial pressure P_i; plasma protein osmotic pressure π_p; and interstitial osmotic pressure arising from escaped plasma protein π_i. The numbers are typical values in mmHg for capillaries in warm human skin [8a] and for human subcutis [11]. Reproduced with permission from [2].

oncotic pressures. The hydraulic pressures are capillary blood pressure (P_c), which drives filtration and derives its energy from the beating of the heart, and interstitial fluid pressure (P_i), which partially opposes capillary pressure. The oncotic pressures are plasma oncotic pressure (π_p), which is the osmotic pressure of plasma proteins and tends to produce absorption of interstitial fluid, and interstitial fluid oncotic pressure (π_i), which partially counteracts the plasma oncotic pressure. Thus Starling's principle can be written in the form

(Filtration rate per unit area A) $\propto$ [(hydraulic pressure difference)−(oncotic pressure difference)]

which can also be written as

$$J_v/A \propto [(P_c - P_i) - (\pi_p - \pi_i)]$$

Upon inserting a proportionality coefficient K_c (the capillary filtration coefficient), a linear equation is obtained

$$J_v/A = K_c [(P_c - P_i) - (\pi_p - \pi_i)] \quad \text{(eqn. 1)}$$

This is often called the Landis–Starling equation.

Capillary structure is not described in detail here, but the reader is reminded that there are three principal kinds of capillary, each with a characteristic range for hydraulic permeability K_c [2]. (i) Continuous capillaries have fairly 'tight' intercellular junctions between their endothelial cells, and hence low K_c values; they occur in skin, lung, muscle, fat and connective tissue, and as 'supertight' capillaries in the brain. (ii) In fenestrated capillaries, the endothelium is perforated by round, 50 nm diameter windows (fenestrae) that are often spanned by a thin membrane which is highly permeable to water. K_c is high in such vessels and they are found in fluid-transferring tissues, such as the kidney, gut mucosa, exocrine glands, synovium, choroid plexus and ciliary body, and also in all endocrine glands. (iii) Discontinuous capillaries have wide, leaky intercellular gaps that allow transfer of red cells. They are found in the liver, spleen and bone marrow.

The key features of the Starling expression were confirmed by micropuncture studies of frog mesenteric capillaries by Landis in 1927, and later for mammalian tissues by Pappen-

heimer and his colleagues using a weighing method to estimate net filtration rate [3]. There have been many subsequent confirmations of the essential truth of the expression [4]. For example, Fig. 5 illustrates a recent study of the Starling principle in synovial joints, where fluid exchange determines the amount of lubricating

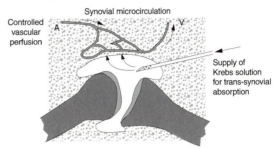

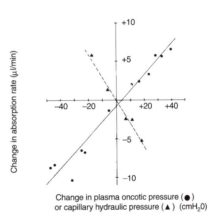

Change in plasma oncotic pressure (●)
or capillary hydraulic pressure (▲) (cmH₂0)

Fig. 5. **Experiment to study fluid exchange in a synovial joint (top) and changes in absorption rate in response to altering capillary pressure or plasma oncotic pressure (bottom)**
(Top) Abbreviations used: A, arterial inflow from a pump; V, venous outflow at controlled pressure. Rate of absorption of saline supplied through the intra-articular cannula was measured by an external drop counter. (Bottom) Changes in rate of absorption of Krebs solution from a joint cavity in response to altering capillary pressure (▲) or plasma oncotic pressure (●) in the perfused synovial microcirculation. The vertical axis is the change in the rate of fluid absorption, so the relationships should pass through zero. The response to oncotic pressure is significantly less steep than that to capillary pressure (ratio 0.7), indicating an osmotic reflection coefficient less than 1. Reproduced with permission from Knight, A.D., Levick, J.R. and McDonald, J.N. (1988) Q. J. Exp. Physiol. **73**, 47–65.

synovial fluid within the joint cavity. The experiment was arranged so that fluid was undergoing absorption from the joint cavity, and the capillary network around the cavity (which contains many fenestrated vessels) was perfused with blood at controlled pressure. When the oncotic pressure of the perfused blood was increased by adding albumin, the rate of absorption of fluid from the joint cavity increased in proportion to the plasma oncotic pressure, showing that fenestrated capillaries behave as semipermeable membranes. When capillary blood pressure was raised, the rate of absorption decreased in linear proportion to the rise in pressure. These results conform with eqn. 1.

The results in Fig. 5 illustrate an additional facet of fluid exchange that is not expressed by eqn. 1. The slope of the osmotic response is not only opposite in sign to the response to capillary pressure, but it is also less steep. This indicates that the osmotic pressure of the plasma protein (albumin in this case) is not exerted fully across the capillary wall. On average, the osmotic response was only 80% as steep as the response to capillary blood pressure, indicating that only 80% of the protein's potential osmotic pressure was actually effective *in vivo*. This is because the capillary wall is an imperfect semipermeable membrane, being slightly leaky to albumin and other plasma proteins. This has, of course, been known for over a century, from the fact that plasma proteins are normal components of peripheral lymph; however, recognition of the implications for fluid exchange awaited the introduction of the osmotic reflection coefficient, by a thermodynamicist called Staverman in 1951.

The reflection coefficient

The osmotic reflection coefficient (usually denoted by σ) is a measure of how effectively a semipermeable membrane discriminates between water and a particular solute, as illustrated in Fig. 6. Its value ranges from 0 to 1 and, in crude terms, this number can be thought of as a measure of the 'goodness' or 'tightness' of the semipermeable membrane; a more formal definition is given later. If the solute radius is bigger than the membrane pore radius, which in turn is big enough to allow water access, then water but not solute can cross the membrane. The solute is then 100% osmotically effective and σ has a value of 1 (Fig. 6, left panel). If, on the other hand, the membrane possesses holes that are far larger than the solute, the solute can access the pore as freely as can the solvent. The membrane is freely permeable to the solute, so no osmotic pressure is exerted (not even if solute is prevented from accumulating on the other side of the membrane) and σ has a value of 0 (see Fig. 6, right panel).

Between these two extremes, there exists a more interesting and physiologically relevant intermediate situation, where the pore is slightly wider than the solute and allows some solute passage, yet is not wide enough to allow solute molecules to access the pore space as freely and fully as the smaller water molecules (Fig. 6, centre panel). The solute now exerts some osmotic pressure across the membrane, but only a fraction of its potential osmotic pressure: this fraction is σ. Thus the osmotic reflection coefficient can be defined formally as 'the ratio of the osmotic pressure actually exerted by a given difference in solute concentration

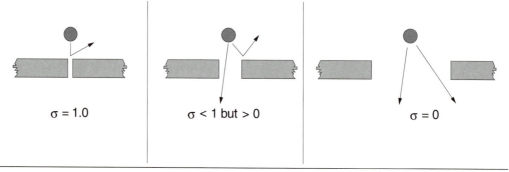

$\sigma = 1.0$ $\sigma < 1$ but > 0 $\sigma = 0$

Fig. 6. **Sketch illustrating how the reflection coefficient σ depends on the ratio of solute radius (a) to pore radius (r)**
In theory, for a cylindrical pore, $\sigma = (1-\phi)^2$, where ϕ, the solute partition coefficient, is given by $(r-a)^2/r^2$. Reproduced with permission from [2].

across the test membrane, to the osmotic pressure that the same difference in concentration would exert across a perfect semipermeable membrane'.

Continuous and fenestrated capillaries are usually found to have plasma protein reflection coefficients in the range 0.8–0.95, although in the very 'tight' brain capillary σ has a value of 1. The reflection coefficient can be determined by comparing changes in filtration rate in response to plasma oncotic pressure changes with those in response to hydraulic pressure changes [9]. An example of this is shown in Fig. 5; here, the change in filtration rate induced by altering plasma oncotic pressure (slope of the oncotic line) is found to be, on average, only 0.8 times that induced by altering capillary blood pressure (slope of hydraulic line), indicating a reflection coefficient of 0.8. The reflection coefficient can also be assessed by analysis of lymph formed at high filtration rates. The most dilute lymph that can be formed reveals the maximum percentage of the plasma protein that can be reflected by the capillary wall, i.e. the reflection coefficient [10] (see also Fig. 13 later). Recently, a novel method based on the transcapillary permeation of radiolabelled plasma albumin has been developed by Renkin and colleagues, and this yielded reflection coefficients of >0.95 in some tissues (for a critical review, see [11]). In view of a widespread misconception that fenestrations are freely permeable to protein, it seems worth emphasizing that fenestrated capillaries as well as continuous capillaries have high reflection coefficients. Measurements like those in Fig. 5 show that fenestral reflection coefficients are similar to those of most continuous capillaries. (The structures responsible for reflection are discussed later in the section entitled Endothelial matrix.)

The reflection coefficient must be entered into the Starling expression, where it serves as a correction factor which establishes the effective oncotic difference across the capillary wall

$$J_v/A = L_p [(P_c - P_i) - \sigma(\pi_p - \pi_i)] \quad \text{(eqn. 2)}$$

A minor point to note in eqn. 2 is the switch from K_c (eqn. 1) to the conventional thermodynamic symbol for the hydraulic conductance of unit area of membrane L_p.

The capillary reflection coefficient is important for several reasons. First, it affects the 'balance' of pressures at each point in the capillary (see later). Secondly, values of σ <1 mean that the capillary wall is permeable to plasma proteins to some degree; the rate of escape of plasma protein into interstitial fluid (and hence π_i) depends in part on σ (see next section). Thirdly, and here is a reason why microcirculationists have been as excited about σ as membrane physiologists have about ionic conductances, σ conveys information about the nature of the pores in the capillary wall. According to a theoretical expression (cited in the legend to Fig. 6), reflection coefficients of 0.8–0.95 for albumin would be produced by cylindrical pores of radius 4.0–5.5 nm, so capillary permeability is classically attributed to pores of equivalent radius 4.0–5.5 nm. It is practically certain, however, that the pores are not cylindrical in reality, and this will be considered further in the final section.

▶ Only part (80–95%) of the osmotic pressure of plasma protein is actually effective at the capillary wall. The osmotic reflection coefficient σ is typically 0.80–0.95 in continuous and fenestrated capillaries.
▶ Reflection coefficients of <1 allow a slow escape of plasma proteins into the interstitial compartment.

The above discussion touched briefly on the escape of plasma protein into interstitium. This influences the size of the interstitial oncotic pressure π_i, and we must next consider the magnitude and functional significance of the extravascular Starling terms.

Magnitude of the extracapillary pressures

Interstitial hydraulic and oncotic pressures (P_i and π_i, respectively) are important determinants of filtration across the capillary wall, although the contrary impression is often conveyed in general physiology textbooks. Indeed, it is common in such accounts to find dismissive statements to the effect that the extravascular Starling terms are small relative to the intravascular pressures, and are therefore negligible. The first half of this statement is true. Plasma oncotic pressure in mammals averages around

25 mmHg (man) to 20 mmHg (laboratory species like rabbit), and mammalian capillary pressure at heart level is typically between 40 mmHg (arterial end of the capillary) and 12–15 mmHg (postcapillary venule): the extravascular pressures are indeed smaller. However, the second part of the statement, implying physiological unimportance, is untrue and seriously misleading, as will be shown below.

Interstitial fluid pressure

The extravascular Starling term that is not attributable to interstitial protein osmotic pressure is traditionally called 'interstitial fluid pressure'. The reason for this somewhat guarded definition is given in the section entitled 'What exactly is being measured?' Most interstitial fluid has a gel-like consistency because a network of fine molecular chains, the glycosaminoglycans (depicted as fine irregular lines in Figs. 7 and 21), permeates the interstitial space and enmeshes the water in tiny spaces. As a result, interstitial fluid does not flow readily, and, despite there being some 12 litres of water in the human interstitial compartment, its pressure is not easy to measure.

Methods

Some of the methods developed to deal with this problem are shown in Fig. 7. Straightforward needle cannulation (see Fig. 7a) is only applicable at special sites or in pathological states where the interstitial compartment contains freely mobile fluid (e.g. normal joint cavity, epidural space, oedematous limb); but micropuncture in conjunction with a servo-nulling pressure measurement system proves successful even in normal interstitium. In the 1960s, Guyton devised the simple but ingenious chronically implanted capsule method as shown in Fig. 7(b). Several weeks are allowed for interstitial fluid and free intracapsular fluid to equilibrate, then the pressure in the cavity is measured via a needle. This resulted in the discovery of 'negative', i.e. subatmospheric, interstitial pressures. The controversy accompanying this discovery triggered a great surge of interest in interstitium and the extravascular Starling terms. Later variants of this method include porous capsules and implanted subcutaneous rings. The wick-in-needle method shown in Fig. 7(c) originated from an idea of Scholander's developed by Aukland, Reed and others [11]. The channels in a multifilamentous

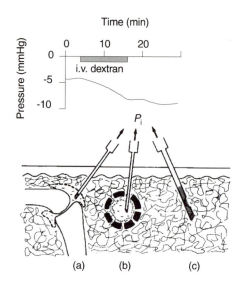

Fig. 7. Methods for measuring interstitial fluid pressure (P_i)
(a) The hypodermic needle method requires a free-fluid space. (b) Guyton's capsule requires chronic implantation. (c) The wick-in-needle method can be applied acutely in man (see text for details). Inset at top: recording of subatmospheric pressure in a synovial cavity (a giant interstitial space); the pressure grows more negative when capillary absorption is induced by an intravenous injection of concentrated dextran solution to raise plasma oncotic pressure.

wick make multiple contacts with the interstitial water and transmit interstitial fluid pressure into the recording system. This method has the advantage of being rapid and applicable in man. There has, in the past, been controversy about the validity of the different methods, particularly the chronic capsule method; however, as Fig. 8 shows, when the capsule, wick and servo-nul micropipette methods are compared in the same species and same tissue at the same time, the results are very similar. The methodological controversy has, therefore, largely abated. (For a detailed methodological review, see [11].)

What exactly is being measured?

The above methods measure an equilibrium pressure, i.e. the pressure at which no flow occurs between the recording device and the interstitial matrix. This state is reached when the free energy level of the water in the recording system is the same as that of the water within the interstitial matrix. The free energy level of water within the gel depends on two factors: the pressure exerted on the gel from outside (approximately atmospheric pressure in the case of soft tissues, such as non-loaded skin), and the gel's osmotic or swelling pressure. The latter requires a few words of explanation. If an excised block of interstitial matrix (e.g. Wharton's jelly) is placed in a beaker of saline, the tissue slowly expands by sucking in water. The swelling is driven by the osmotic pressure of the interstitial glycosaminoglycans, which arises chiefly from a Gibbs–Donnan ionic distribution caused by fixed negative charges on the glycosaminoglycan chains. The Starling term 'interstitial fluid pressure' is thus less simple than might first appear, but this does not matter as far as the effect on capillary filtration rate is concerned (eqn. 2).

Magnitude of interstitial fluid pressure

As the inset in Fig. 7 shows, interstitial fluid pressure is commonly subatmospheric. This is often called a 'negative' pressure, meaning in relation to the atmosphere. (In strict physical terms, there is of course no such thing as negative pressure, since pressure is a force per unit area arising from molecular bombardment.) If

plasma oncotic pressure is increased, e.g. by infusing a concentrated solution of albumin or dextran intravenously, as in the experiment of Fig. 7, a transient absorption of fluid from the interstitial space occurs and interstitial fluid pressure falls to a more subatmospheric level. Interstitial pressure is thus a dynamic variable dependent on microvascular filtration rate, as well as being a factor determining the filtration rate (eqn. 2).

In many tissues (e.g. skin, subcutis, lung, synovium, some relaxed muscles and epidural space), interstitial fluid pressure is subatmospheric and quite small: 0 to –2 mmHg in Fig. 8. In some encapsulated tissues (e.g. kidney, bone marrow), however, supra-atmospheric pressures occur, and large pressures develop in contracting skeletal muscle and myocardium. Pressures are also supra-atmospheric in inflamed tissues, in cancer tissue and in oedema, because interstitial pressure is related to the degree of hydration of a tissue.

In non-encapsulated tissues, like skin and subcutis, the interstitial pressure–volume relationship or compliance curve is highly non-linear (sigmoidal). P_i is a steep function of vol-

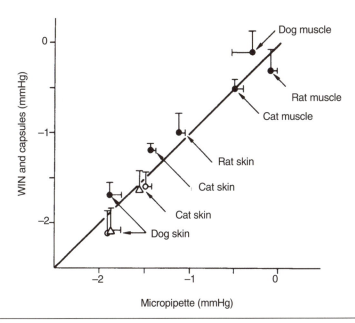

Fig. 8. Measurements of interstitial fluid pressure in skin and relaxed muscle by the wick-in-needle (WIN, ●), porous capsule (△) or hollow capsule (○) method

Each result is compared with a simultaneous servo-nul micropipette measurement. Reproduced with permission from [11].

ume at subatmospheric pressures because changes in water content alter the glycosaminoglycan concentration of the interstitium, and hence the component of interstitial pressure that is attributable to glycosaminoglycan osmotic pressure. When tissue fluid volume has increased by about 50–100%, however, there are no further significant changes in glycosaminoglycan os-motic pressure, because it has fallen virtually to zero. P_i now becomes nearly independent of hydration and attains a plateau a few millimetres of Hg above atmospheric pressure, reflecting a slight elastic compression by investing tissue, such as skin. Interstitial compliance is thus quasi-infinite in moderate oedema. Only with extreme oedema formation does P_i rise much further, owing to the stress exerted by grossly distorted surrounding tissues. Changes in P_i with hydration probably contribute just a little (a few millimetres of Hg) to the buffering of filtration rate, and hence to the 'safety margin' against oedema, in tissues such as subcutis and lung [11,12]. The changes can be greater, however, in encapsulated tissues, such as the kidney and some skeletal muscle compartments.

Interstitial oncotic pressure

Interstitial oncotic pressure is the osmotic pressure of interstitial fluid caused by plasma proteins that have escaped into the interstitium across the capillary wall. Interstitial oncotic pressure is generally bigger than P_i; indeed, it often approaches venous pressure in size i.e., about 10 mmHg.

Methods

Interstitial oncotic pressure is not easy to measure because interstitial fluid is not readily aspiratable. A common early approach was to collect pre-nodal lymph on the assumption (probably valid) that its composition is representative of nearby interstitial fluid. In recent years, direct, acute sampling of human subcutaneous interstitial fluid has been made possible by the development of the implanted wick method of Aukland and colleagues [13]. A saline-soaked multifilamentous wick is stitched through the subcutis and left to equilibrate with the surrounding interstitial fluid for an hour. The wick is then pulled out, its fluid extracted by centrifugation and analysed.

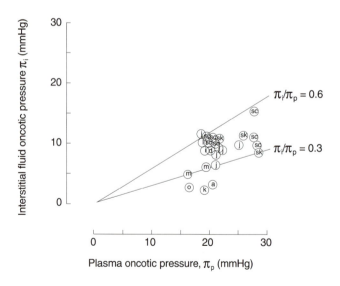

Fig. 9. Magnitude of interstitial fluid oncotic pressure in a wide variety of mammalian tissues

The values are plotted against the corresponding plasma oncotic pressure and the guidelines delineate ratios of 0.3 and 0.6. Abbreviations used: a, intestinal mucosa during water absorption; d, dermis; i, intestine; j, joint; k, kidney; l, lung; m, mesentery; o, omentum; sc, subcutis; sk, skeletal muscle. Data assembled from various authors. Reproduced with permission from [13a].

Magnitude

Interstitial oncotic pressures determined with the wick and other methods in a wide variety of tissues and species are compared with plasma oncotic pressure in Fig. 9. As the guidelines indicate, the interstitial oncotic pressure is typically 30–60% of the plasma oncotic pressure in muscle, skin and subcutis, tissues that together account for nearly half the body weight in a lean person. Lower values are found in tissues in which there is net absorption of water into capillaries (kidney, gut mucosa) and higher values in tissues with leaky discontinuous capillaries (liver, bone marrow, spleen). Values of 30–60% plasma level can by no means be considered negligible and, in the next section, their substantial physiological importance is described.

> ▶ Interstitial fluid pressure is subatmospheric in some tissues (e.g. subcutis, lung, synovium) and supra-atmospheric in others (e.g. kidney). Its size varies with hydration and hence with capillary filtration rate.
> ▶ Interstitial oncotic pressure is 30–60% of plasma oncotic pressure in many tissues. It is thus relatively large and contributes substantially to an imbalance of Starling pressures across the capillary wall.

Reassessment of the filtration–absorption diagram

Traditional view

Direct micropuncture of frog mesenteric and human nailfold capillaries by Landis in the 1930s proved that mean capillary pressure is very close to plasma oncotic pressure. In man this is true at heart level, though capillary pressure below heart level exceeds oncotic pressure due to the effect of gravity. Human skin capillary pressure is high (35–40 mmHg) in the arterial segment of the capillary and falls progressively to a near venous level (12–15 mmHg) at the venular end of the capillary. It was probably this observation that gave rise to the popular concept illustrated in the left-hand panel of Fig. 10. It was thought that in the steady state fluid filters out of the arterial segment of the mammalian capillary, because P_c (35 mmHg) exceeds π_p (25 mmHg), and is largely reabsorbed into the venous segment, because π_p (25 mmHg) exceeds P_c (12–15 mmHg), the small residuum being carried away as lymph. π_p changes little along the axis of a well-perfused continuous capillary, because the filtration fraction is <1%. This is essentially the view put forward in the influential review by Landis and Pappenheimer [3]. Interstitial terms were thought to be small at that time.

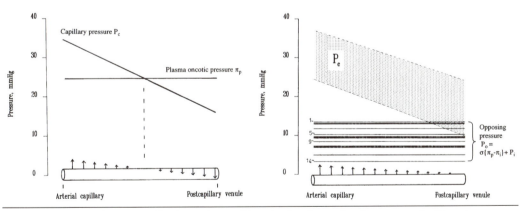

Fig. 10. Gradient of pressure P_c along the capillary bed at heart level compared with net pressure opposing filtration

(Left) Plasma oncotic pressure π_p is about midway between arterial and venous capillary pressures. If these were the only factors involved in fluid exchange, flow might be as sketched below (traditional filtration–absorption diagram). (Right) Stippled zone shows spread of P_c for a range of tissues and mammalian species. Horizontal lines show P_0, the true net pressure opposing capillary pressure, namely $\sigma\,(\pi_p - \pi_i) + P_i$. 1, rabbit omentum; 2, dog skeletal muscle; 3, cat mesentery; 4, rabbit mesentery; 5, rat mucosa in resting state; 6, human subcutis; 7, cat dermis; 8, rat subcutis; 9, rabbit subcutis; 10, rabbit shoulder; 11, rat tail; 12, rabbit elbow; 13, rabbit knee; 14, dog lung. In every individual tissue P_0 is less than P_c, even at the postcapillary venule. The resulting fluid-exchange pattern is sketched below. Data assembled from various authors. Reproduced with permission from [13a].

Starling sums with modern extravascular measurements incorporated

The filtration–reabsorption concept was developed at a time when the extravascular Starling pressures were thought to be small, and therefore relatively unimportant, and the osmotic reflection coefficient was taken to be effectively 1. When later measurements of interstitial hydraulic pressure, interstitial oncotic pressure and the capillary reflection coefficient are taken into account, however, a different picture emerges, as shown in the right-hand panel of Fig. 10. Here, the capillary pressure and plasma oncotic pressure are exactly the same as in the left-hand panel, but the incorporation of a slightly negative interstitial pressure, substantial interstitial oncotic pressure and a reflection coefficient of <1 raises the sum of Starling pressures at every point along the capillary, in the direction of filtration. The shift is so large that there is no longer a net absorption force in the venous segment of the capillary. The chief reason for the loss of the putative downstream net reabsorption force is that the extravascular forces, far from being negligible, are together of a similar magnitude to the difference between plasma oncotic pressure and postcapillary venular pressure, which is the maximum potential absorptive force. The picture that emerges for a well-perfused capillary is one of filtration throughout the vessel, gradually dwindling and reaching almost nil near the venular end. This applies to skin, subcutis, relaxed muscle, synovial joints, omentum and intestinal smooth muscle; in each tissue the sum of the measured Starling forces indicates a small net filtration force in the downstream segment of the exchange vessels, at or below heart level.

Effect of gravity on Starling sums

The caveat raised earlier concerning heart level is important in man. Direct microcannulation of skin capillaries in human fingers and toes (Fig. 11) shows that capillary pressure increases below heart level, owing to the effect of gravity on the arterial and venous blood columns serving the capillary bed (see Chapter 5, Fig. 10). It will be noticed that there is a progressive shift of the capillary pressure line away from the arterial pressure line in Fig. 11 as the tissue becomes dependent, with the result that capillary pressure increases by less than arterial or venous pressure. The relative position of the capillary pressure, in between arterial and

venous pressure, is set by the ratio of precapillary to postcapillary resistances, and the protective shift away from arterial pressure seen in Fig. 11 arises from a graded arteriolar constriction with dependency. In daily life, limb motion must reduce capillary pressure to some degree, since the calf muscle pump reduces venous pressure in the feet. Even so, it is obvious that most capillaries below heart level do not have a reabsorbing segment; and in man in the upright position, the majority of the microcirculation is below heart level. As Fig. 11 shows, capillary pressure changes little above heart level, probably because of venous collapse and arteriolar dilatation, so the above argument does not apply in reverse to the upper part of the body. Gravity has little direct effect on interstitial fluid pressure because of the gel-like state of the fluid.

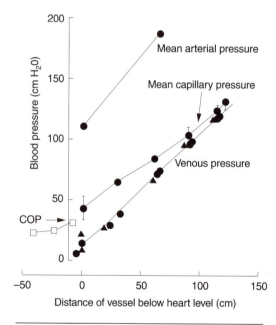

Fig. 11. Vascular pressures in man as a function of vertical distance below or above heart level

*Capillary pressure in skin measured by direct micropuncture. COP indicates human plasma colloid osmotic pressure. Arteriolar constriction with dependency (the veni-arteriolar response) is revealed by the progressive shift of capillary pressure away from arterial pressure and towards venous pressure. Results taken from Landis, E.M. (1930) Heart **30**, 209–238 (open symbols) and [8a] (closed symbols).*

When absorption does occur

Simple arithmetic based on measured Starling pressures thus provides no support for the traditional view that there is a near balance between filtration and reabsorption along the length of a well-perfused capillary in the steady state, either at heart level, above or below it. This is only one of several reasons for questioning the traditional view: there are also theoretical and experimental reasons. Before going into these, however, it is important to note that absorption of interstitial fluid by capillaries can unquestionably occur, given the right circumstances. These fall into two classes: (i) tissues that are specialized for sustained fluid absorption (intestinal mucosa, renal peritubular microcirculation and lymph nodes) and (ii) in other tissues, transient absorption follows acute capillary hypotension, whether caused by physiological arteriolar vasoconstriction or by a pathological state such as hypovolaemic hypotension (see Chapter 5) [14]. The situation in specialized absorbing tissues will be discussed later: the transient absorption after a sudden fall in capillary pressure is considered first.

Fig. 12 depicts the sequence of events during capillary hypotension. The left-hand panel shows the normal steady state, just as in the right-hand panel of Fig. 10, namely dwindling filtration throughout a well-perfused capillary at heart level. If the arteriole feeding this vessel constricts, due to sympathetic or humoral stimuli, capillary pressure falls (centre panel) and the vessel shifts into a state not unlike that traditionally depicted as normal, namely upstream filtration (at a reduced rate) and downstream absorption (Fig. 12b). Absorption can outweigh filtration because the hydraulic permeability of the venular capillary wall is considerably higher than that of the arterial segment — a phenomenon called the 'arterio-venous gradient of permeability'. In addition, in some tissues, the number of venous capillaries exceeds the number of arterial capillaries, due to branching.

Fig. 12(b) contains no surprises, but what is of considerable interest (and this has been confirmed experimentally, see Fig. 15 later) is that this situation is not sustained in vessels with a finite permeability to plasma protein ($\sigma < 1$). As time passes, the selective absorption of water by the venous segment causes the concentration of interstitial protein around the absorbing region to increase (because the extravascular protein is largely reflected by the

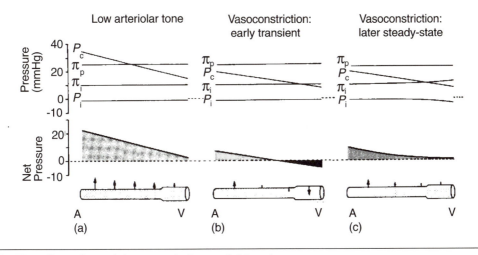

Fig. 12. **The effect of arteriolar constriction on fluid exchange**

From top: axial gradients of capillary pressure, P_c; plasma oncotic pressure, π_p; interstitial oncotic pressure, π_i; interstitial fluid pressure, P_i; and their sum, the net pressure (with correction of oncotic pressures for $\sigma = 0.9$). Sketch below shows direction of fluid exchange from arteriolar beginning of capillary (A) to its venular end (V). (a) Well-perfused capillary; values are the same as in Fig. 4. (b) Immediately after arteriolar vasoconstriction; transient absorptive state due to reduced capillary pressure. (c) Eventual steady state if vasoconstriction is maintained; downstream absorption abolished by rise in interstitial oncotic pressure and fall in interstitial hydraulic pressures. Reproduced with permission from [2].

endothelium). This produces an upturn in the π_i line downstream (see Fig. 12, right panel). Also, interstitial fluid pressure begins to fall due to interstitial dehydration. Both these changes oppose fluid absorption. The greater the amount of fluid absorbed, the greater the counteracting changes in π_i and P_i, until, eventually, these changes fully offset the local absorptive pressure ($\pi_p - P_c$) and absorption ceases. Thus absorption is transient in the class (ii) situation (see above). This transience is a vivid illustration of the importance of extravascular factors.

> ▶ Summation of the four Starling terms, using measured values and correcting osmotic terms by σ, does not support the traditional filtration–reabsorption concept of fluid balance in most tissues. The venular segment is in a state of slight filtration in the steady state, not absorption.
> ▶ Absorption can occur as a transient event when capillary pressure falls, e.g. after arteriolar vasoconstriction or hypovolaemia. The absorption is transient, except in tissues specialized for fluid absorption.

There is both experimental and theoretical evidence for the above sequence of events. First, let us consider the evidence that the concentration of plasma protein in interstitial fluid varies with capillary filtration rate in the way just described.

Interstitial oncotic pressure as a dynamic variable dependent on filtration rate

Understanding the factors that govern the concentration of plasma protein in interstitial fluid is crucial to understanding fluid exchange, because interstitial protein concentration determines interstitial oncotic pressure. The concentration of protein in interstitial fluid (C_i), relative to that in plasma (C_p) (ratio C_i/C_p) is an inverse function of capillary filtration rate. This is illustrated in Fig. 13. Here, filtration rate in the dog paw was varied by means of venous congestion and estimated by the resulting lymph flow in the steady state. C_i was indicated by the protein concentration in the paw lymph C_L. When filtration rate was increased,

C_L fell, and at high filtration rates it approached a limiting value which, according to theory, equals $1 - \sigma$. Albumin, for example, reached a limiting dilution of about 0.15 or 15% of plasma level, indicating a reflection coefficient of 0.85. Fig. 13 shows results for three plasma proteins of increasing size, albumin (67 kDa), γ-globulin (150 kDa) and fibrinogen (330 kDa), and it can be seen that the bigger the protein molecule, the lower the C_L/C_p ratio, i.e. the greater the degree of mole-

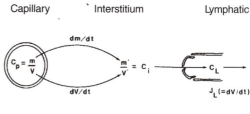

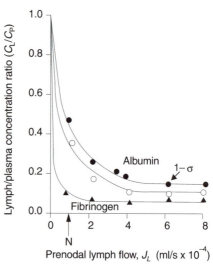

Fig. 13. **Effect of net microvascular filtration rate, measured as prenodal lymph flow J_L, upon the lymph/plasma concentration ratio C_L/C_P for various plasma proteins**
*Lymph concentration is used as a convenient measure of interstitial concentration. Three proteins of increasing size are shown, namely albumin (67 kDa), γ-globulin (50 kDa) and fibrinogen (330 kDa). Their limiting dilution at high flows equals $1 - \sigma$; σ increases with molecular size. Filtration rate was varied by adjusting venous pressure. N indicates normal value. Dog paw results from Renkin et al. (1977) Microvasc. Res. **14**, 191. (Top) Mechanism underlying the effect of filtration rate on protein concentration, as described in the text. Reproduced with permission from [2].*

cular sieving and the bigger the reflection coefficient. This kind of approach has been widely used to estimate reflection coefficients and capillary pore sizes [10].

The mechanism underlying the inverse relation is sketched at the top of Fig. 13. C_i is mass m' divided by volume V'. In a dynamic system, this ratio depends on the mass of protein arriving by diffusive and convective transport across the capillary wall in a given time (transport rate dm/dt) divided by the volume of water arriving by filtration over the same period (filtration rate dV/dt): $C_i = (dm/dt)/(dV/dt)$. A rise in filtration rate increases the water transfer more than the protein transfer, owing to partial reflection of the protein. As a result, the ratio m'/V' (concentration) falls. This in turn reduces π_i. This is an interesting situation because *interstitial oncotic pressure is a determinant of filtration rate, yet filtration rate is a determinant of interstitial oncotic pressure.* This mutual interdependence has two important consequences, namely buffering of filtration rate and transience of absorption states, as described below.

(1) Buffering of filtration rates

Changes in π_i act as an important osmotic buffer against excessive filtration rates [11,12]. The way this operates is illustrated in Fig. 14. The top panel of the figure is essentially a copy of the curve in Fig. 13 except that the ordinate has been transformed from concentration to oncotic pressure. If filtration rate rises, interstitial oncotic pressure falls, so the difference between plasma and interstitial oncotic pressures, i.e. the absorption pressure $(\pi_p - \pi_i)$, increases (point C). This will, in turn, tend to oppose the rise in filtration rate that is causing the change. How then can we decide by how much filtration rate and absorption pressure change, i.e. what determines the particular combination of values when the tissue is in a steady state?

A graphical analysis provides a useful insight into how the effects of filtration rate on absorption pressure, and absorption pressure on filtration rate together establish a steady state (Fig. 14, lower panel). The abscissa is filtration rate and the ordinate is oncotic absorption pressure. The curved line shows how increases in filtration rate raise the absorption pressure; the curve is simply read off the results in the upper panel. The continuous straight line

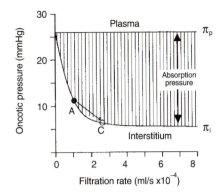

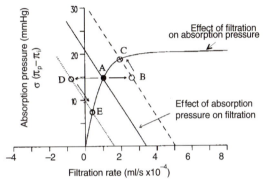

Fig. 14. A graphical analysis of the steady state for capillary fluid exchange

(Top) Effect of filtration rate on interstitial oncotic pressure and absorption pressure (plasma oncotic pressure minus interstitial oncotic pressure). This difference is shown as a striped zone. Point A represents a typical normal value. Calculated from data in Fig. 13. (Bottom) Curve shows oncotic absorption pressure from top panel plotted as function of filtration rate. Increases in filtration rate raise the absorption pressure; the curve is simply read off the results in the top panel. The continuous straight line represents the Starling equation relation for the dog paw, namely filtration rate as a function of absorption pressure when the driving pressure $(P_c - P_i)$ is fixed; the intercept on the pressure axis equals $P_c - P_i$. The convention of placing the dependent variable on the ordinate was reversed for the Starling line to allow it to be shown on the same plot. The point of intersection of the two lines at A gives the only stable filtration rate, i.e. the steady-state value. The dashed line is the Starling relationship when $P_c - P_i$ is raised by 10 mmHg; note the buffering of filtration rate between B and C. The dotted line is the relationship when $P_c - P_i$ is reduced to 10 mmHg; note the initial absorption (D), reverting to slight filtration in the steady state (E). Adapted and reproduced with permission from [13a].

represents the Starling equation (eqn. 2) and shows how increases in oncotic absorption pressure reduce the filtration rate, if the hydraulic pressure drop across the capillary wall, $P_c - P_i$, is constant. The usual convention regarding the axis for the independent variable (normally the abscissa) has been reversed for the Starling line to allow it to be shown on the same plot. The Starling line and the absorption pressure curve intersect at point A, and this is the only point at which a given pair of filtration rate and absorption pressure values lies simultaneously on both curves. This is, therefore, the only stable situation, i.e. the steady state, where the effects of filtration rate on absorption pressure exactly matches the effect of absorption pressure on filtration rate. By way of illustration, consider a filtration rate a little higher than point A. This would raise the absorption pressure (move it up the curve from A, to the right); but, as the Starling line shows, a rise in absorption pressure would reduce the filtration rate (a move up the straight line, from point A, to the left) and the situation would be unstable. Filtration rate and absorption pressure would readjust until the only stable combination, point A, is re-established. It is, therefore, the intersection of the Starling line and absorption pressure curve which determines steady-state fluid exchange, for a given pressure drop across the capillary wall.

[If the reader finds this aspect of fluid exchange difficult upon first acquaintance, it may help to point out that the approach is analogous to that used by Guyton to determine steady-state cardiac output from the intersection of a venous return curve and Starling law of the heart curve. It can also be compared with that used by respiratory physiologists to determine steady-state ventilation from the intersection of a PCO_2–ventilation response curve and Loeschke metabolic hyperbola (effect of ventilation on PCO_2).]

The graphical analysis of the steady state proves useful when considering the osmotic buffering of filtration rate in the face of oedemagenic challenges. If capillary pressure rises for any reason, such as raised venous pressure in heart failure, the Starling line is shifted upwards, since its intercept on the ordinate is $P_c - P_i$ (see Fig. 14, lower panel); this follows from substituting $J_v = 0$ into eqn. 2. Immediately after raising capillary pressure, the oncotic pressures are unchanged, so there is an

initial rise in filtration rate to point B. The filtration rate then attenuates, however, because the raised filtration rate increases the oncotic absorption pressure (oncotic buffering), until finally a new steady state is reached at point C. Starling himself clearly recognized the significance of dynamic changes in interstitial protein concentration; in his classic paper of 1896 he wrote, 'With increased capillary pressure there must be increased transudation, until equilibrium is established at a somewhat higher point, when there is more dilute fluid in the tissue spaces and therefore a higher absorbing force to balance the increased capillary pressure'.

The buffering capacity of this mechanism is limited by the magnitude of normal interstitial oncotic pressure, because the latter can at best fall only as far as zero. The mechanism is particularly powerful in the lung, because here the interstitial protein concentration is normally 66–69% of that in plasma and the interstitial oncotic pressure is 16–20 mmHg. This provides one of the 'safety factors against oedema' [12].

(2) Transience of venular fluid reabsorption

The interstitial protein dilution/concentration curve is important for a second reason. It buffers fluid absorption and, after some time, it causes absorption to cease altogether (see Fig. 14, lower panel). When capillary pressure falls, the capillary is initially tipped into absorption (point D). As a result, interstitial protein concentration gradually rises. Therefore, after the initial maximum reabsorption rate (point D), there is a progressive fall in absorption pressure and absorption rate, until finally the capillary shifts back into slight filtration (point E). Again, the steady state is given by the intersection of the line and curve. The pulmonary system is an excellent example of a tissue that normally operates close to point E. In the lungs P_c is much smaller than π_p; nevertheless, there is continuous formation of lymph, i.e. capillary filtration, because π_i rises to a high level [8].

Fluid absorption is thus generally a self-cancelling process. Sustained fluid reabsorption is not possible in vessels with even a minor permeability to plasma protein unless the tight coupling between interstitial protein concentration and filtration rate is somehow broken (as in tissues specialized for fluid absorption; see later). Again, Starling seems to have recognized this, stating in 1896, 'With diminished capillary pressure there will be an osmotic absorption of salt solutions from the extravascular fluid, until this becomes richer in proteids; and the difference between its [proteid] osmotic pressure and that of the intravascular plasma is equal to the diminished capillary pressure. Here then we have the balance of forces necessary to explain the accurate and speedy regulation of the quantity of circulating fluid'.

> ▶ Interstitial protein concentration increases when filtration rate falls, and decreases when filtration rate rises, in capillaries permeable to protein.
> ▶ Raised filtration rates are buffered by the ensuing fall in interstitial oncotic pressure. The latter raises the oncotic absorption pressure across the capillary wall, i.e. plasma oncotic pressure minus interstitial oncotic pressure.
> ▶ Interstitial fluid absorption is a self-cancelling process in most tissues because interstitial oncotic pressure rises during fluid absorption, progressively reducing the absorption pressure.

The above analysis is based on whole-tissue results for interstitial protein, such as those in Fig. 13. Can we accept it as a valid argument against sustained downstream reabsorption in individual venular capillaries (forgetting, for a moment, the arithmetical evidence against this in Fig. 10)? The 'proof' is not absolute, but it would require a rather special anatomical arrangement to avoid the conclusion that local venular absorption is also a self-cancelling process. For such an absorption to be sustained, it would be necessary for the stream of filtrate from the arterial segment to be directed past the venular segment en route to the lymphatic system, so as to flush the perivenular interstitium and dissipate the accumulating perivenular protein. There is no evidence for this kind of flow pattern in most tissues.

Experimental studies: the non-linear relationship of filtration rate to capillary pressure in the steady state

The argument that sustained downstream absorption is not sustainable, except under spe-

cial circumstances, was developed on theoretical grounds by Michel [4]. Direct experimental evidence was provided by Michel and Phillips [15] in a study of fluid movement across segments of individual capillaries in the frog mesentery — which might be considered to be the microcirculationist's equivalent of the giant squid axon. Pressure was varied in capillaries perfused with a slightly hyperoncotic solution. If capillary pressure was reduced below plasma oncotic pressure immediately after commencing the perfusion, fluid absorption was observed, as shown in Fig. 15 (this corresponds with a shift from A to D in Fig. 14). But, when the perfusion was maintained for 2–5 min at low capillary pressure, and the measurement of fluid exchange repeated, absorption no longer occurred, even at very low capillary pressures. Absorption dwindled to zero or even reversed to slight filtration despite capillary pressure being lower than plasma oncotic pressure — rather as in the lungs, and as in point E of Fig. 14. Over the 2–5 min perfusion period, during which there was absorption at first, plasma protein presumably accumulated in the interstitium around the capillary, because there was no filtration stream to wash it away and diffusional dissipation was too slow to do so. Consequently, π_i increased and P_i may have fallen a little too. This abolished the absorption process in the perfused capillary segment, as predicted by mathematical theory [4] and by the equivalent graphical analysis in Fig. 14(b). The results provide an experimental demonstration of the great importance of labile extravascular forces.

Because the interstitial Starling terms are a function of filtration rate and, therefore, of capillary pressure, the relationship between capillary pressure and filtration in the steady state is not a linear one at low pressures. The effect is most marked when P_c is near to or less than π_p. The relationship is linear at high capillary pressures because the interstitial terms are then not far from zero and are, therefore, relatively stable. It is thus no coincidence that the steady-state relationship for the single frog capillary (Fig. 15, filled circles) is very similar to the relationship between left atrial pressure, a determinant of pulmonary capillary pressure, and the rate of oedema formation in the lung [16].

The evolution of our understanding of fluid exchange has been nicely summarized by Renkin (Fig. 16). Beginning with the primitive or 'amoeboid' form of the Starling equation and

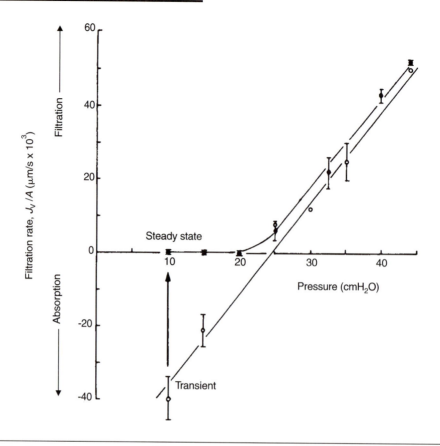

Fig. 15. Filtration rate in a segment of frog mesenteric capillary (J_v/A, ordinate) perfused at various capillary pressures (abscissa)

Perfusate oncotic pressure was 32 cmH₂O, which is higher than normal for a frog. When fluid exchange was measured immediately after starting the perfusion (○), low capillary pressures caused fluid absorption. If, however, perfusion was maintained for 2–5 min before fluid exchange was measured (allowing time for interstitial forces to alter), no absorption was seen at low capillary pressures (●). Reproduced with permission from [15].

the idea of forces in balance [Fig. 16 (1) and (2)], Landis's work on the frog led to an expression for filtration rate (3). With the introduction of the reflection coefficient (4), the way was prepared for the recent evolution of Michel's monster: the non-linear expression (5) [4,17]. Here, π_i has disappeared as an independent variable but is present in the guise of a non-linear function of π_p and the Peclet number. The latter is a dimensionless parameter that represents the relative rate of convective transport [$J_v(1-\sigma)$] to diffusional transport [PA (permeability × surface area)] for plasma protein. This expression describes a non-linear relationship between steady-state filtration rate J_v and capillary pressure P_c, like the curve in Fig. 15, and it shows the role of finite protein permeability (PA) and

the reflection coefficient in causing the non-linearity.

To recapitulate, three lines of evidence indicate that for a wide range of tissues filtration prevails downstream in the steady state, and hence that the traditional filtration–absorption diagram is not a generally valid representation of fluid exchange along the capillary–venular axis in the steady state. The three lines of evidence are (i) summation of all four Starling pressures measured in a given tissue (Fig. 10 and Fig. 11); (ii) graphical or theoretical analyses that take account of the rise in interstitial protein concentration when filtration rate declines (Fig. 14 and Fig. 16); and (iii) direct experiments on single capillary segments (Fig. 15).

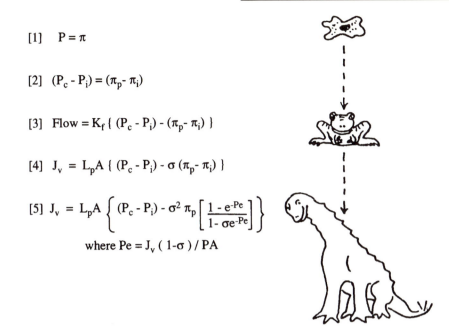

$$[1] \quad P = \pi$$

$$[2] \quad (P_c - P_i) = (\pi_p - \pi_i)$$

$$[3] \quad \text{Flow} = K_f \{ (P_c - P_i) - (\pi_p - \pi_i) \}$$

$$[4] \quad J_v = L_pA \{ (P_c - P_i) - \sigma (\pi_p - \pi_i) \}$$

$$[5] \quad J_v = L_pA \left\{ (P_c - P_i) - \sigma^2 \pi_p \left[\frac{1 - e^{-Pe}}{1 - \sigma e^{-Pe}} \right] \right\}$$

$$\text{where } Pe = J_v (1-\sigma) / PA$$

Fig. 16. **The evolution of the Starling expression**
This illustrates the progression from the most primitive form of the Starling principle to the form derived by Michel in 1984 (neglecting the non-linearity of the relationship of C_i to π_i). Perhaps the dinosaur indicates that the evolutionary process is still not complete; for example, P_i is not a truly independent variable but depends partly on J_v. Reproduced with permission from [17].

Non-steady states: potential anti-oedema role of vasomotion

Increasingly, it seems important to take account of the fact that in tissues with active arteriolar vasomotion, such as skin and resting muscle, the capillaries may actually spend a considerable fraction of their time in non-steady states. The physiological 'norm' may be a continual alternation between filtration, as the terminal arteriole dilates, and transient reabsorption as the terminal arteriole constricts, i.e. a constant switching from state A (in Fig. 12) to state B and back, under the influence of vasomotion. The periods of constriction and transient fluid absorption could help prevent the development of tissue oedema. Relatively little is known about this temporal aspect of fluid exchange but it would help to explain why mean blood pressure in the exchange vessels is typically about 7 mmHg lower when calculated indirectly from net fluid filtration rate divided by wall conductance L_p (a procedure that averages P_c over space and time), than when measured by direct micropuncture in a well-perfused capillary. Indeed, the ratio of lymph flow to capillary filtration coefficient indicates that the net filtration pressure across the capillary walls, averaged over space and time, is ≤1 mmHg in many tissues [11]. It must be admitted that the details of how a given tissue achieves interstitial fluid balance are often still poorly understood.

Tissues where sustained fluid absorption occurs

But what about tissues where sustained absorption of fluid by the microcirculation does occur, i.e. lymph nodes, gut mucosa during intestinal water absorption, and renal peritubular capillaries? What special property allows these tissues to maintain an absorptive state, despite the above results and theory? The answer, illustrated in Fig. 17, is that the interstitial space in each of these tissues has a fluid input that is independent of local capillary filtration. This breaks the tight linkage that normally exists between π_i and transcapillary flow; that is, Fig. 14 does not apply in such tissues. The independent source of interstitial water is the afferent lymph flow in the case of lymph nodes, the water absorbed from the gut lumen in the case of the mucosa, the renal tubular absorbate in the case of the kidney, and the artificial infusate in the experiment illustrated in Fig. 5. The fluid washes through the interstitium in each case, and the portion of it that is not absorbed by the capillaries flushes any escaped plasma proteins away from the pericapillary space and into the lymphatic system. With interstitial protein accumulation thereby prevented, there is no bar to sustained capillary absorption. It has to be added that the details of this process are still not well understood, especially in the inner renal medulla, which appears to lack a lymphatic system.

▶ Measurements of fluid exchange in single capillaries confirm that absorption cannot be sustained when capillary pressure is reduced below plasma oncotic pressure if σ is <1. This is the normal situation in the lung.

▶ Arteriolar vasomotion may be important in producing repeated states of transient fluid absorption in some systemic tissues; however, in many tissues, achievement of fluid balance is still not fully understood.

▶ In the gut mucosa, renal peritubular system and lymph nodes, sustained capillary absorption is possible because a separate fluid input into the interstitium (e.g. water from gut or tubule lumen) flushes the interstitium and prevents interstitial oncotic pressure from rising during absorption.

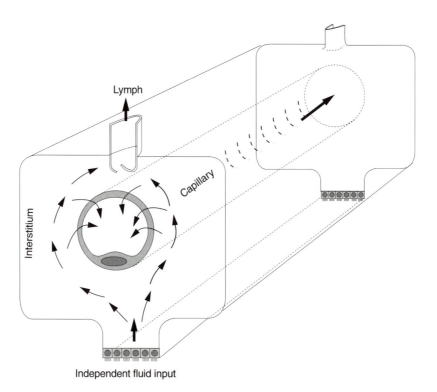

Fig. 17. Fluid exchange in a tissue capable of sustained absorption into capillaries (gut mucosa, renal cortex peritubular system)

The interstitium is flushed by part of the epithelial absorbate, namely the portion that passes into the lymphatic system, and this prevents interstitial accumulation of escaped plasma protein. In the case of a lymph node, where the microcirculation is also capable of sustained absorption, the epithelium in the sketch would be replaced by an afferent lymphatic. Reproduced with permission from [13a].

Fibrous matrices inside and outside the capillary

The account so far has concentrated on developments in our understanding of the Starling principle of fluid exchange, without paying much attention to the physical nature of the pores in the capillary wall that permit the flow of water and largely reflect the plasma proteins. The issue of resistance outside the capillary wall has also been ignored so far. However, in the 1980s there were developments in both these areas. First, a new theory concerning the fundamental nature of capillary porosity, the 'fibre matrix' theory, was developed by Curry and Michel in 1980 [9,18]; they attributed the capillary's molecular selectivity to a network of fibrous molecules or glycocalyx coating the endothelial cells. Secondly, it has been found that in some tissues the hydraulic resistance of the interstitium surrounding the capillary is great enough to affect fluid exchange in the steady state. Interstitial resistance is caused by a matrix of fibrous molecules, the glycosaminoglycans. Thus the endothelial cell can be regarded as a cellular sandwich between two fibrous matrices with differing properties (or three, bearing in mind the basement membrane). The remainder of this chapter reviews briefly these aspects. The interstitial matrix is considered first.

Extravascular matrix and hydraulic resistance

The interstitium is criss-crossed by a molecular network of long-chain polymers (glycosaminoglycans, proteoglycans and glycoproteins; Fig. 21) that are entangled in and partially bound to a scaffolding of collagen fibrils [19]. Depending on the concentration of the biopolymers in a particular tissue, the mesh size in the molecular network can be so small that it creates considerable resistance to flow [20]. In circumstances where the hydraulic resistance of the capillary wall itself is low — as in fenestrated capillaries and inflamed capillaries, for example — interstitial resistance can be a significant fraction of the resistance of the overall fluid pathway. This can reduce capillary filtration rate by imposing a significant gradient of interstitial fluid pressure between capillary and 'sink' (e.g. lymphatic or joint cavity), which raises interstitial fluid pressure around the capillary.

An example of a tissue where capillary wall resistance is low (owing to fenestrations) and interstitial resistance is relatively high is the synovial lining of a joint, which is shown in sketches in Fig. 5 and Fig. 18. The relationship between capillary pressure and rate of absorption of fluid from the joint cavity was touched on earlier (see Fig. 5). The slope of this relationship depends on the net conductance of the combined interstitial pathway and capillary wall (conductance being the reciprocal of resistance). It was found that the thickness of interstitium intervening between the joint cavity and the capillary fenestrations could be reduced by stretching the lining (achieved by raising intraarticular pressure): this is illustrated in Fig. 18 (top panel). The same process also caused the hydraulic conductance of the combined interstitium–endothelium layer to increase, as shown in the lower panel of Fig. 18. This finding is most readily explained if the interstitium normally accounts for a significant fraction (about half) of the hydraulic resistance between the joint cavity and capillary plasma, and this fraction decreases as the layer gets thinner. Synovium is like many other tissues specialized for fluid exchange (e.g. exocrine grands) in that it possesses fenestrated capillaries. The high hydraulic permeability of fenestrae enhances the importance of the interstitial resistance, which lies in series with capillary wall resistance. Interstitial resistance is probably relatively less important in tissues with continuous capillaries, whose walls offer a relatively higher resistance. Whenever capillary wall resistance is low, however, as in fenestrated capillaries and inflamed vessels [9], the resistance of the extravascular matrix may significantly affect steady-state fluid movement.

Endothelial matrix and capillary permeability

There is little doubt that water and small solutes cross the capillary wall predominantly via the intercellular junctions in continuous capillaries, and via fenestrations in fenestrated capillaries. But difficulties have long been experienced in simultaneously describing hydraulic permeability, solute permeability and reflection coefficient results by a pore theory based on cylindrical or slit pores penetrating the capillary wall [5,6]. In addition, it has long been known that a thin layer of fibrous molecules, namely negatively charged sialoglycoproteins and gly-

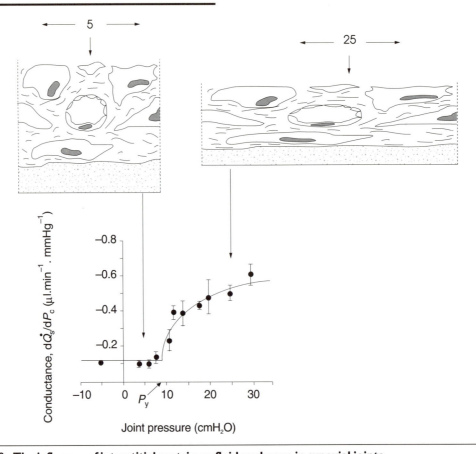

Fig. 18. The influence of interstitial matrix on fluid exchange in synovial joints

*Some key features of synovium are shown in the upper sketches, i.e. fenestrated capillaries separated from the joint cavity (top) by interstitium-filled intercellular spaces. Morphometry shows that when joint pressure is raised from 5 to 25 cmH₂O the tissue stretches and the interstitial 'barrier' between capillary and cavity grows thinner. The effect on the hydraulic conductance of the combined interstitium–capillary wall pathway from joint cavity to plasma is shown in the graph. Conductance was determined from the slope of plots such as Fig. 5 (dashed line) at a series of joint pressures. Q_S is trans-synovial flow in the rabbit knee. Reproduced with permission from Knight, A. D. and Levick, J.R. (1985) J. Physiol. **360**, 311, and Levick, J.R. and McDonald, J.N.. (1989) J. Physiol. **419**, 493.*

cosaminoglycans, coats the internal surface of the capillary, including the entrance to the intercellular junctions and the surface of fenestrations, as illustrated in Fig. 19. Curry and Michel suggested in 1980 that this endothelial glycocalyx might influence permeation and resolve the quantitative difficulties in reconciling experimental results with pore theory [18]. Their idea was that the filamentous glycocalyx molecules might be sufficiently densely packed to form a network with a mesh size small enough to reflect most macromolecules, yet wide enough to allow the passage of water and small solutes into the underlying intercellular slits and fenestral diaphragm pores. Although this concept had qualitative precedents, Curry and Michel suggested a theoretical framework that allowed quantitative predictions of fibre matrix effects and this, coupled with growing experimental evidence in its favour, has given the fibre matrix theory considerable vitality.

Evidence relating to the fibre matrix theory was considered in a recent Review Lecture to the Physiological Society by Michel [9] and some of this evidence is reproduced in Fig. 20. The hydraulic permeability (L_p) of the capillary wall was determined from the slope of the relationship between capillary pressure and filtra-

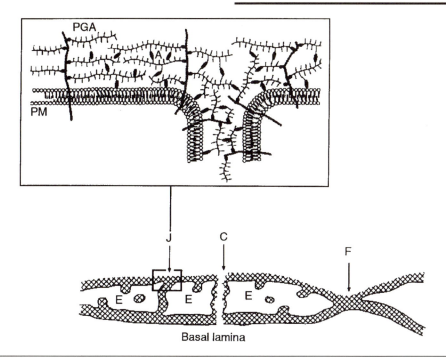

Fig. 19. Fibre matrix model of capillary permeability

For details, see text. Abbreviations used: E, endothelium; F, fenestra; C, transcellular channel (a macromolecular escape route, very infrequent); J, junctional cleft between adjacent cells; PGA, proteoglycan fibre of glycocalyx; PM, plasmalemma membrane. There is evidence that albumin normally binds via its positively charged arginine groups to the PGA-fixed negative charges, ordering the network and reducing permeability (the protein effect). Reflection coefficients are governed by mesh size and regularity. Permeability depends also on the number and dimensions of the intercellular clefts and fenestrae. Reproduced with permission from [6] and [9].

tion rate. When there was no protein in the intravascular perfusate, capillary permeability was abnormally high and σ was low. When the perfusate contained even a small concentration of albumin, the permeability (slope) and σ quickly reverted to normal — a dramatic effect known rather mundanely as 'the protein effect'. This had been known for a long time, but in the experiment illustrated in Fig. 20 the protein effect was induced not by albumin, but by a positively charged protein, cationized ferritin. When this was added to the perfusate, the effect on the slope was dramatic. Electron microscopy was then used to locate the site of the cationized ferritin in the capillary wall. As the electron micrograph in Fig. 20 shows, the positively charged ferritin bound to the glycocalyx. Native ferritin, which has no net positive charge, failed to exert the protein effect (failed to restore normal permeability) and also failed to bind to the glycocalyx. These findings strongly implicate the glycocalyx as a determi-

nant of capillary permeability. It is worth stressing that the fibre matrix theory is not a rival to the pore theory but a supplement to it; the area and length of the 'open' part of the junctional cleft underneath the glycocalyx remain important factors influencing permeability. The recognition that the endothelial cell-surface coat, whose density and composition is presumably controlled by intracellular mechanisms, is an important determinant of permeability, raises distant but tantalizing vistas of the pharmacological manipulation of permeability, perhaps with eventual therapeutic implications.

The other chief structure conferring a high water conductance on some endothelial cells is the fenestra or fenestration, as noted in the Introduction. Most fenestrations, except in renal glomerular capillaries, are bridged by a thin, osmophilic diaphragm, and each diaphragm is penetrated by about 14 pores. It was widely assumed, in the past, that the diaphragm

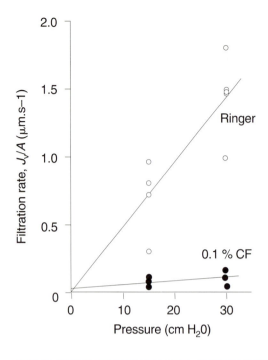

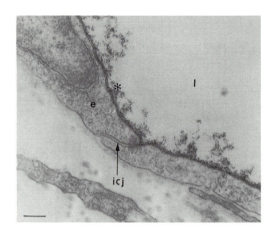

Fig. 20. Effect of protein on capillary permeability
(Left) Filtration rate versus pressure in a single capillary (frog mesentery) perfused initially with protein-free Ringer solution (○) then with cationized ferritin (●). The slope L_p was reduced on average by 70% by the cationized ferritin. Albumin has a similar effect but native ferritin has no significant effect. (Right) The electron micrograph shows that cationized ferritin (tiny black dots) *binds to the endothelial glycocalyx (*). Abbreviations used: e, endothelium; l, capillary lumen. Native ferritin does not bind to the endothelium. Note that the labelled glycocalyx covers the entrance to the intercellular junction (icj). Reproduced with permission from Turner, M., Clough, G. and Michel, C.C. (1983) Microvasc. Res. **25**, 205.*

was the main source of resistance to fluid and solute transfer across fenestrae, but this view has been challenged recently.

An analysis of permeability data in relation to fenestral geometry indicated that the diaphragm is far too thin to offer significant resistance if it contains as much as a single pore. (The 4–5 nm thick diaphragm is, in fact, thinner than an albumin molecule.) Put another way, the fenestral pathway is more than an order of magnitude less permeable than it would be if the diaphragm were the sole obstacle in the pathway and contained even one small pore [21]. It seems, therefore, that other, thicker structures must exist in the fenestral pathway and dominate resistance to exchange (as has long been recognized in the renal glomerulus). The obvious candidates for this role are the glycocalyx and/or basement membrane.

▶ A network of fibrous molecules coats the endothelial cell surface. This 'glycocalyx' probably governs the reflection coefficient and contributes to resistance to fluid movement through intercellular clefts and fenestrae.
▶ A network of fibrous molecules just outside the capillary wall, the basement membrane, probably also contributes to the resistance to fluid exchange in fenestrated capillaries.
▶ A network of fibrous molecules in the interstitium (interstitial glycosaminoglycan matrix) can contribute to the overall resistance to fluid circulation in certain circumstances, e.g. synovial lining, inflamed capillaries.

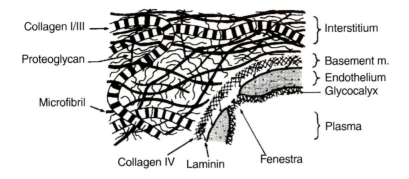

Fig. 21. The microvascular–interstitial exchange pathway viewed as three fibrous matrices in series

(i) Endothelial glycocalyx (overlying fenestral pores, as shown here, or intercellular clefts in continuous capillaries); (ii) basement membrane (collagen type IV, laminin, glycosaminoglycan); and (iii) interstitium (collagen fibrils, type I/III fibrils, type VI microfibrils, proteoglycans, hyaluronan, glycoproteins). The thickness, density, regularity and charge of each matrix determine its permeability. Reproduced with permission from [22].

Today's perspective

Fig. 21 summarizes a current view of capillary permeability. It actually depicts a fenestrated capillary in synovial interstitium, but a similar picture could be drawn for a continuous capillary by replacing the fenestra with an intercellular cleft and the joint cavity by a lymphatic vessel. According to this viewpoint, fluid exchange is a process of flow across three fibrous matrices arranged in series, each of different biochemical composition and density. Fluid must first cross the endothelial fibrous matrix, which probably determines the reflection coefficient of the capillary wall. The fluid then crosses the capillary wall, either via intercellular clefts of limited area (relatively high resistance) or the fenestral diaphragm (very low resistance). The area and length of these pathways influence permeability. Next, the fluid must traverse a second fibrous matrix, the basement membrane. Finally, it flows through a third fibrous matrix, the interstitium, to reach its destination, which might be the lymphatic system, a joint cavity or a secretory acinus. The extravascular circulation of fluid can thus be conceptualized as a process of flow across a set of different fibrous matrices arranged in series. This seems a far cry from the notion of simple pores, a featureless interstitial 'bath' and negligible intersti-

tial Starling pressure that so many textbooks of physiology still portray.

Finally, it must be pointed out that many exciting recent developments in capillary physiology are not covered here. A particularly active, important area, involving endothelial cell biology, concerns the regulation of capillary permeability by endothelial intracellular Ca^{2+}. Inflammatory mediators, such as histamine, cause an influx of extracellular Ca^{2+} through calcium-conducting channels in the endothelial cell wall, as well as release of stored Ca^{2+}. The ensuing activation of the endothelial cytoskeleton by Ca^{2+} probably mediates gap formation and permeability increases. This field has been reviewed recently [23].

References

References [9, 11 and 17] are essential reading.

1. Adair, T.H. and Guyton, A.C. (1983) Modification of lymph by lymph nodes. Am. J. Physiol. **245**, H616–622

2. Levick, J.R. (1991) Solute transport between blood and tissue and Circulation of fluid between plasma, interstitium and lymph. In An Introduction to Cardiovascular Physiology, pp. 117–170, Butterworth–Heineman, London

3. Landis, E.M. and Pappenheimer, J.R. (1963) Exchange of substances through the capillary walls. In Handbook of Physiology, Section 2, (Hamilton, W.F. and Dow, P., eds.), pp. 961–1034, Am. Physiol. Soc., Bethesda

4. Michel, C.C. (1984) Fluid movements through capillary walls. In Handbook of Physiology, Section 2, Volume IV

(Renkin, E.M. and Michel, C.C., eds.), pp. 375–409, Am. Physiol. Soc., Bethesda

5. Crone, C. and Levitt, D.G. (1984) Capillary permeability to small solutes. In Handbook of Physiology, Section 2, Volume IV (Renkin, E.M. and Michel, C.C., eds.), pp. 411–466, Am. Physiol. Soc., Bethesda

6. Curry, F.E. (1986) Determinants of capillary permeability: a review of mechanisms based on single capillary studies in the frog. Circ. Res. **59**, 367–380

7. Knox, P. and Pflug, J.J. (1983) The effect of the canine popliteal node on the composition of lymph. J. Physiol. **345**, 1–14

8. Staub, N.C., Flick, M., Perel, A., Landolt, C. and Vaughan, T.R. (1981) Lung lymph as a reflection of interstitial fluid. In Tissue Fluid Pressure and Composition (Hargens, A.R., ed.), pp. 113–124, Williams and Wilkins, Baltimore

8a. Levick, J.R. and Michel, C.C. (1978) The effects of position and skin temperature on the capillary pressures in the fingers and toes. J. Physiol. **274**, 97–109

9. Michel, C.C. (1988) Capillary permeability and how it may change. J. Physiol. **404**, 1–29

10. Taylor, A.E. and Granger, D.N. (1984) Exchange of macromolecules across the microcirculation. In Handbook of Physiology, Section 2, Volume IV (Renkin, E.M. and Michel, C.C., eds.), pp. 467–520, Am. Physiol. Soc., Bethesda

11. Aukland, K. and Reed, R.K. (1993) Interstitial-lymphatic mechanisms in the control of extracellular fluid volume. Physiol. Rev. **73**, 1–78

12. Taylor, A.E. and Townsley, M.I. (1987) Evaluation of the Starling fluid flux equation. News Physiol. Sci. **2**, 48–52

13. Kramer, G.C., Sibley, L., Aukland, K. and Renkin, E.M. (1986) Wick sampling of interstitial fluid in rat skin: further analysis and modification of the method. Microvasc. Res. **32**, 39–49

13a. Levick, J.R. (1991) Capillary filtration–absorption balance reconsidered in light of dynamic extravascular factors. Exp. Physiol. **76**, 825–857

14. Lanne, T. and Lundvall, J. (1989) Very rapid net transcapillary fluid absorption from skeletal muscle and skin in man during pronounced hypovolaemic circulatory stress. Acta Physiol. Scand. **136**, 1–6

15. Michel, C.C. and Phillips, M.E. (1987) Steady-state fluid filtration at different capillary pressures in perfused frog mesenteric capillaries. J. Physiol. **388**, 421–435

16. Guyton, A.C. and Lindsey, A.W. (1959) Effects of elevated left atrial pressure and decreased plasma protein concentration on the development of pulmonary edema. Circ. Res. **7**, 649–657

17. Renkin, E.M. (1986) Some consequences of capillary permeability to macromolecules: Starling's hypothesis reconsidered. Am. J. Physiol. **250**, H706–710

18. Curry, F.E. and Michel, C.C. (1980) A fibre-matrix model of capillary permeability. Microvasc. Res. **20**, 96–99

19. Bert, J.L. and Pearce, R.H. (1984) The interstitium and microvascular exchange. In Handbook of Physiology, Section 2, Volume IV (Renkin, E.M. and Michel, C.C., eds.), pp. 521–548, Am. Physiol. Soc., Bethesda

20. Levick, J.R. (1987) Flow through interstitium and other fibrous matrices. Q. J. Exp. Physiol. **72**, 409–438

21. Levick, J.R. and Smaje, L.H. (1987) An analysis of the permeability of a fenestra. Microvasc. Res. **33**, 233–256

22. Levick, J.R. (1989) Synovial fluid exchange: a case of flow through fibrous mats. News Physiol. Sci. **4**, 198–202

23. Curry, F.E. (1992) Modulation of venular microvessel permeability by calcium influx into endothelial cells. FASEB J. **6**, 2456–2466

Glossary

Anterograde
Travelling in the same direction as the nerve impulse. In neurophysiological terms it usually refers to transport within nerve fibres. In sensory nerves, transport would be toward the central nervous system, whereas in motor fibres transport would be toward the periphery. It is the opposite of **retrograde** in which case the transport is in the reverse direction. Transport often makes use of axoplasmic flow within the nerve fibres.

Apnoea
The term used when there is a total cessation of breathing.

Aortic bodies
Glomus tissue in the walls of the aortic arch which has chemosensitive properties. The activity of the cells increases when the arterial blood PO_2 or pH falls, or when its PCO_2 increases. The tissue is supplied by sensory fibres which travel to the **nucleus tractus solitarius** in the **aortic nerve**, a branch of the vagus Xth nerve.

Autoregulation
In some vascular beds the blood flow is maintained constant even when there are changes in the perfusion pressure. This is known as autoregulation or pressure autoregulation. It is due in part to the inherent properties of the arterial smooth muscle cells (see also **Myogenic** response).

Bradycardia
Slowing of the heart beat caused by, for example, activation of vagal efferent fibres supplying the sinu-atrial node (pacemaker).

Bulbospinal neurone
A neurone whose cell body lies in the brainstem (bulb) and whose axon descends to the spinal cord where it terminates.

Cardioexcitatory
An influence in which the activity of the heart (usually heart rate) is increased. The opposite effect: **cardioinhibitory**.

Carotid bodies
Glomus tissue found in the bifurcation of the carotid artery which has chemosensitive properties. It has an extremely high blood flow per gram of tissue. The activity of the cells increases when the arterial blood pH or PO_2 falls or when its PCO_2 increases. The tissue is supplied by sensory fibres which travel to the **nucleus tractus solitarius** in the **carotid sinus nerve**, a branch of the glossopharyngeal (IXth cranial) nerve.

Carotid sinus
A thin-walled region of the internal carotid artery close to the bifurcation of the carotid artery. The carotid sinus arterial baroreceptors (mechanoreceptors which monitor changes in the arterial pressure) are found in the wall of the sinus. They are supplied by sensory fibres which travel to the **nucleus tractus solitarius** in the **carotid sinus nerve**, a branch of the glossopharyngeal (IXth cranial) nerve.

Central inspiratory drive
A measure of the overall neural output of the various groups of inspiratory neurones in the brainstem. It can be measured as the activity of the **phrenic nerve**, the motor nerve supplying the diaphragm.

Decerebration
The removal of the rostral parts of the brain. The amount of tissue removed can vary. If only the cerebral cortex is removed this is termed **decortication**. Usually more tissue than the cortex is removed, the section being made between the colliculi in the midbrain. The **hypothalamus** may or may not be intact, depending on the exact level and angle of the decerebration.

Depressor response
Refers to a fall in mean arterial pressure. It is the opposite of a **pressor response** when mean arterial pressure is increased.

Diuresis
An increased rate of production of urine by the kidneys (see also **Natriuresis**).

Dorsal vagal motor nucleus
A group of neuronal cell bodies in the dorsomedial part of the brainstem. One origin of vagal motor (parasympathetic) fibres supplying the lungs, heart and upper digestive tract (see also **Nucleus ambiguus**).

Eupnoea
The minute ventilation of an individual at rest (see also **Hyperpnoea** and **Apnoea**).

Hyperaemia
An increase in blood flow to a tissue: may occur as a result of an increased metabolic rate of the tissue (see active, functional or **Metabolic hyperaemia**) or following a period of ischaemia (reactive hyperaemia).

Hypercapnia
An increase in the arterial PCO_2.

Hyperplasia
An increase in cell number which can sometimes accompany **hypertrophy**.

Hyperpnoea
Occurs when minute ventilation is increased, for example during exercise (see also **Eupnoea** and **Apnoea**).

Hypertension
A persistently elevated level of arterial blood pressure above the normal range for the age group of the individual. May be caused by several different mechanisms.

Hypertrophy
An increase in the size of a cell. It usually refers to muscle cells and the increase in their size evoked in response to exposure to increased work loads. It is distinct from an increase in cell number (see **Hyperplasia**) which can sometimes accompany hypertrophy.

Hypotension
Arterial blood pressure below the normal range.

Often occurs as a result of haemorrhage.

Hypovolaemia
A reduction in the circulating blood volume.

Hypoxia
A reduction in the availability of oxygen to the peripheral tissues. This may be due to a low arterial blood PO_2 (**hypoxic hypoxia**), low systemic or local blood flow (**stagnant hypoxia**), reduced oxygen-carrying capacity of the blood (**anaemic hypoxia**) or cellular metabolic poisoning (**histotoxic hypoxia**).

Intermediolateral cell column
A longitudinal column of neurones located in the lateral horn of the spinal cord. It includes the cell bodies of **sympathetic preganglionic neurones**. Their axons leave the spinal cord via the ventral roots and make synapses with the cell bodies of **sympathetic postganglionic neurones** in ganglia in the sympathetic chain or in collateral sympathetic ganglia.

Ischaemia
Literally a checking or a deficiency of blood supply to an organ or tissue. It occurs when the blood flow to a tissue or organ is insufficient to maintain the normal metabolism and results in hypoxia, hypercapnia and accumulation of other metabolites. It usually results from a total or partial obstruction of a vessel by, for example, a blood clot (thrombosis). Strictly speaking, ischaemia is also

present when a tissue is artificially perfused with a physiological fluid (e.g. Krebs–Ringer) rather than blood.

Meninges
The brain and spinal cord are covered by three membranous layers which help protect it. The thick outer layer is the dura mater, inside which is the thinner arachnoid. The thin pia mater adheres to the surface of the brain and spinal cord. The space between the arachnoid and pia mater is filled with cerebrospinal fluid.

Metabolic hyperaemia
An increase in blood flow to an organ or tissue as a result of increased activity of the tissue. The increased activity results in production of vasodilator metabolites and thus increased vascular conductance. Also known as **active** or **functional hyperaemia**.

Muscle pump
When skeletal muscles contract the deep veins are compressed and blood expelled from them each time the muscle contracts. Venous valves prevent any retrograde flow and the expelled blood is therefore directed toward the heart. This mechanism is the muscle pump and is an important aid to maintaining central venous pressure and ventricular filling pressure during muscular contraction.

Myogenic response
Raising the pressure inside a blood vessel tends to distend the vessel. However, most

arterioles then respond by constricting back to their original diameter, or even smaller. This myogenic response is a response to stretch of the smooth muscle cells comprising the arteriolar wall. It is important in allowing the blood flow in some vascular beds to remain constant even when arterial pressure changes (*autoregulation*, or pressure autoregulation)

Natriuresis

This is an increase in the rate at which sodium is excreted from the body in the urine. It can be calculated from the urine flow rate multiplied by the urine sodium concentration.

Nucleus ambiguus

A diffuse collection of neuronal cell bodies in the ventrolateral part of the brainstem. An origin of motor fibres (somatomotor and parasympathetic) to the pharynx and palate, the upper and lower airways, the heart, lungs and oesophagus (see also **Dorsal vagal motor nucleus**).

Nucleus tractus solitarius

A sensory nucleus in the dorsomedial part of the brainstem. It can be subdivided into various subnuclei, including the medial, lateral and commissural subnuclei. It receives and integrates sensory information travelling in the VIIth (facial), IXth (glossopharyngeal) and Xth (vagus) cranial nerves. This sensory input arises from gustatory, airway, pulmonary, cardiac, gastric, intestinal and other abdominal receptors.

Reflex gain

In a reflex an applied stimulus will evoke an appropriate response. In negative feedback control the response tends to minimize the evoked change and return the variable back to its initial level. If a stimulus–response relationship is constructed, the maximum slope of this relationship is the **gain** or **sensitivity** of the reflex. The absolute level of the variable which the reflex is tending to maintain is called its **set point**. In certain circumstances, the set point may be altered to a higher or lower value. This is termed **resetting** of the reflex.

Respiratory sinus arrhythmia

The speeding up of the heart rate during inspiration as a result of decreased vagal inhibitory action on the sinu-atrial node. The response is partly a reflex due to activation of pulmonary stretch receptors but can occur even when lung inflation is prevented. In this case it is due to interactions in the brainstem between the activity of respiratory neurones (**central inspiratory drive**) and vagal motor neurones.

Reticular formation

A diffuse network of small neurones and fibres forming the 'core' of the brainstem. It is found in the most primitive vertebrates but is maintained throughout phylogenetic development. The constituent cells are not organized into easily identifiable groups on the basis of their histology or connections.

Rostral ventrolateral medulla

A group of neurones in the ventrolateral part of the rostral brainstem. At least some are **bulbospinal**, sending axons to the **intermediolateral cell column** of the spinal cord where sympathetic preganglionic neurones are located, i.e. they can be thought of as **'presympathetic'** interneurones. They are thought to provide one source of the **sympathetic vasomotor tone**. They are distinct from, but receive input from, the neurones in the **caudal ventrolateral medulla** which do not project to the intermediolateral cell column.

Sympathoexcitatory

An influence which increases activity in one or more sympathetic nerves. It is the converse of **sympathoinhibitory**.

Tachycardia

Increase in heart rate. Can be the result of one or more of the following: decreased parasympathetic (vagal) or increased sympathetic nervous activity or the release of adrenaline from the adrenal medulla acting at the sinu-atrial node (pacemaker).

Vagus nerve

The Xth cranial nerve. A mixed nerve containing both afferent (sensory) fibres and efferent (motor) fibres. It supplies the upper and lower airways, the lungs, heart and upper digestive tract. Sensory fibres terminate in the **nucleus tractus** solitarius. Motor fibres have their origin in the two vagal motor nuclei, the **dorsal vagal nucleus** and the **nucleus ambiguus.**

Vascular conductance
When a fluid flows along a rigid tube the flow (Q) is proportional to the pressure gradient between the inlet (P_1) and the outlet (P_2), i.e. $Q \propto P_1 - P_2$. Adding a proportionality constant (K) will produce an equation describing flow:

$$Q = K \cdot (P_1 - P_2)$$

K is the conductance of the tube. In blood vessels the equivalent is known as the vascular conductance. At constant perfusion pressure, changes in conductance produce parallel changes in flow in the vascular bed. **Vascular conductance** is the reciprocal of the **vascular resistance.**

Vascular resistance
This is the reciprocal of **vascular conductance** (see above). Thus, at constant flow, changes in resistance produces changes in the perfusion pressure of the vascular bed.

Vasomotor tone
A measure of the amount of constriction of resistance vessels. This constriction depends in part upon the level of activity in the sympathetic vasoconstrictor nerves that supply the vessels: the **sympathetic vasomotor tone.** In addition, after removal of the nerve supply, vessels exhibit a certain level of **basal tone** which is an intrinsic property of the vascular smooth muscle itself.

Venous occlusion plethysmography
A non-invasive technique which can be used to measure the blood flow to a limb. The limb is either sealed in an airtight container or a strain gauge is fixed around its greatest circumference. The venous outflow is temporarily occluded by inflating a cuff around the limb to a pressure higher than venous pressure. The initial rate of change in the volume of the limb then reflects the arterial blood flow into the limb.

Index

Absorption of interstitial fluid, 139
Adenosine, 120
Adenosine antagonist, 121
ADH (see Antidiuretic hormone)
Adrenaline, 42
Airway receptor, 9
Amygdala, 11, 46
Anaesthesia, 25, 43
Angiotensin II, 79
ANP (see Atrial natriuretic peptide)
Antidiuretic hormone, 79
Aortic body, 24
Aortic nerve, 65
Arousal, 70
Arterial baroreceptor, 5, 10, 21, 29, 68, 108
Arterial chemoreceptor, 10, 107
Arterial pressure, 51, 61
Arteriolar resistance vessel, 114
Arteriole, 124
Atrial natriuretic peptide, 79
Atrial receptor, 81, 82
Atropine, 42

Baroreceptor, 5, 10, 21, 29, 68, 81, 108
Baroreceptor pathway, 11
Baroreceptor reflex, 12, 44, 69, 109
Behavioural alerting, 39
Behavioural control system, 75
Blood volume, 77
Bradycardia, 24, 88
Brainstem, 1
Breath-hold diving, 27
Bronchodilator drug, 32
Buffering of filtration rate, 141

Capillary
    hydraulic permeability of wall, 148
    passage of solute across wall, 127
    regulation of permeability, 151
    relationship of pressure to filtration rate, 143
    structure, 131

Carbon dioxide, 51, 67, 117
Cardiac afferent fibre, 57
Cardiac arrest, 32
Cardiac C-fibre, 21
Cardiac output, 93
Cardiac vagal activity, 64
Cardiac vagal motoneurone, 9, 19, 20, 30
Cardiac ventricular receptor, 90
Cardiovascular neurone, 110
Cardiovascular reflex, 5, 10, 18, 68, 86
Cardiovascular system, 96
Carotid body, 24
Carotid body chemoreceptor, 21, 30
Carotid sinus nerve, 30, 65
Cellular uptake and degradation mechanism, 122
Central command, 100
Central chemosensitivity, 51
Central inspiratory neuronal drive, 17
Cerebral blood flow, 66
Cerebral vessel, 118
Chemoreceptor, 10, 21, 30, 43, 68, 69, 107
Compliance, 85
Conditioning, 43
Cortisol, 83

Defence response, 13
Denervation, 69
Desynchronized sleep, 61
Diving response, 27, 30
DLH (see D-L-Homocysteic acid)
Dorsal root, 73
Dynamic exercise, 94

EEG (see Electroencephalogram)
Electroencephalogram, 61
Emersion from water, 31
Emotional stress, 41
Endothelial cell, 123
Endothelial intracellular calcium, 151
Endothelial matrix, 147
Endothelium, 124

Exercise, 47, 93, 94
Extracapillary pressure, 133
Extracellular fluid, 77
Extracellular hydrogen ion concentration, 118
Extravascular matrix, 147

Face immersion, 29, 30
Fainting, 55
Filtration–absorption diagram, 137
Filtration rate
    buffering, 141
    glomerular, 80
    relationship to capillary pressure, 143
Flow-induced dilatation, 123
Fluid balance, 78
Frontal cortex, 55
Functional hyperaemia, 113

Gastro-oesophageal reflux, 33
Glomerular filtration rate, 80
Glycine, 49
Gravitational stress, 86
Gravity, 87, 138
Guyton's capsule, 134

Habituation, 52
Haemorrhage, 57, 87
Head-up tilting, 87
Heart beat, 34
Heart rate, 63
D-L-Homocysteic acid, 47
Hydraulic permeability of capillary wall, 148
Hydrostatic pressure, 77
Hypercapnia, 69
Hypertension, 53
Hypertrophy, 54
Hypotension, 86
Hypothalamic defence area, 12, 45
Hypothalamus, 11, 22, 37
Hypoxia, 25, 44, 70

IML (see Intermediolateral cell column)
Implanted wick method, 136
Inorganic phosphate, 120
Input to respiratory neurone, 22
Integrative mechanism, 28
Intermediolateral cell column, 3
Interstitial fluid
    absorption, 139
    pressure, 134
Interstitial oncotic pressure, 136, 140
Interstitial potassium ion concentration, 119
Interstitial resistance, 147
Interstitium, 147

Intestinal water absorption, 145
Intracellular fluid, 77
Irreversible shock, 88, 90
Isometric exercise, 94

Joint afferent, 97
Juxtaglomerular apparatus, 80

Lactate, 117
Loop of Henle, 80
Lower body negative pressure, 57
Lung inflation, 23
Lymph, 128
Lymph node, 145

Mayer wave, 17
Mediator of metabolic vasodilatation, 115
Metabolic activity, 67
Metabolic control system, 75
Metabolic vasodilatation, 115
Metaboreceptor, 110
Motor command, 100
Motor cortex, 47
Muscle
    afferent, 97
    blood flow, 106
    chemoreflex, 105
    pump, 85
    receptor, 98
    vasoconstriction, 63
    vasodilatation, 38

NA (see Nucleus ambiguus)
Nitric oxide, 123, 124
NO (see Nitric oxide)
Non-linear expression, 144
NTS (see Nucleus tractus solitarius)
Nucleus ambiguus, 2
Nucleus tractus solitarius, 2
Nucleus raphe obscurus, 74

Ondine's curse, 76
Osmolarity, 120
Oxygen, 70, 115

$PaCO_2$, 67
PaO_2, 70
Parasympathetic nerve, 8, 81
Paraventricular nucleus, 4
Periaqueductal grey, 46
Peripheral vasoconstriction, 24
pH, 117
Phasic period of sleep, 62
Plasma volume, 127

Playing dead, 41
Posturally induced hypotension, 86
Potassium, 98, 118, 119
Preganglionic neurone, 4, 8
Presympathetic neurone, 4, 23
Primate, 41
Prostaglandin, 122
Protein effect, 149
Proximal tubule, 80
Pulmonary receptor, 9, 18
Pulmonary reflex, 17

Rapid eye movement, 61
Reactive hyperaemia, 113
Reflection coefficient, 132
Reflex from larynx, 33
Regulation of blood volume, 77–90
Regulation of capillary permeability, 151
REM (see Rapid eye movement)
Renal peritubular capillary, 145
Renal sympathetic nerve, 65
Renin, 79, 83
Respiratory drive, 9
Respiratory modulation
    of cardiovascular reflex, 18
    of excitatory cardiac motoneurone, 20
    of presympathetic
    neurone, 23
Respiratory neurone, 22, 110
Respiratory reflex, 69
Respiratory sinus arrhythmia, 16
Restoration of heart beat, 34
Reticular activating system, 72
Reversible shock, 90
Rostral ventrolateral medulla, 4, 11
RVLM (see Rostral ventrolateral medulla)

Saffan anaesthesia, 25
Sensitivity of baroreceptor reflex, 109
Sensitization, 52
Sham rage, 37
Shock, 88, 90
SIDS (see Sudden infant death syndrome)
Sino-aortic denervation, 69
Sleep, 61–76
Slowly adapting pulmonary-stretch receptor, 10
Sodium, 78
Spinal cord, 73, 74
Starling sum, 138
Starling's principle, 130
Stress, 41, 86

Sudden infant death syndrome, 33
Sustained fluid absorption, 145
Sympathetic activity, 3, 4, 11, 41
Sympathetic cholinergic fibre, 41
Sympathetic nerve, 81
Sympathetic outflow, 22
Sympathetic preganglionic neurone, 4
Sympathoexcitatory neurone, 7
Synchronized sleep, 61
Systemic hypoxia, 25, 44

Thoracic duct, 129
Tissue acidosis, 117
Tonic period of sleep, 62
Traube–Hering wave, 17
Trigeminal nerve, 30
Trigeminal receptor, 29

Vagal preganglionic neurone, 8
Vagal tone, 9
Vascular capacitance, 78, 84
Vascular resistance, 85
Vasoactive product, 114
Vasoconstriction, 24, 88
Vasodilatation, 38, 88
Vasodilator metabolite, 89
Vasodilator nerve, 38, 89
Vasodilator neurotransmitter, 124
Vasomotion, 145
Vasomotor centre, 1
Vasomotor neurone, 110
Vasomotor tone, 3, 6
Vasopressin, 79
Vasovagal syncope, 55, 88
Vein, 84
Venous pooling, 87
Venous potassium ion, 119
Ventral medulla, 49
Ventricular afferent, 58
Venular fluid reabsorption, 142

Wick-in needle method, 134

Physiology titles from Portland Press

Interstitium, Connective Tissue and Lymphatics

R K Reed, N G McHale, J L Bert, C P Winlove and G A Laine

This book offers new perspectives on the inter-relationship of the structure and function of the interstitium, and the formation and propulsion of the lymph. It updates and summarizes our knowledge of regulatory mechanisms at the genomic and cellular levels in relation to these areas of tissue physiology, including presentation and discussion of new experimental approaches, investigations of new systems, and an appreciation of new mechanisms involved with connective tissue physiology.

It is split into four parts: structure; physical properties; lymphatic function; and integrated function of tissue systems.

1 85578 073 9 Hardback   356 pages   £75.00/US$120.00   July 1995

Clinical Pulmonary Hypertension

A H Morice, *Royal Hallamshire Hospital, Sheffield, UK*

Contents: The normal pulmonary circulation, J M B Hughes; Pulmonary hypertension in childhood: clinico-pathological correlations, S G Haworth; Pathology of adult pulmonary hypertension, S Stewart; Investigation and diagnosis of pulmonary hypertension in adults, C M Oakley; Pulmonary hypertension in chronic obstructive pulmonary disease, D Dev and P Howard; Thromboembolic pulmonary hypertension, L G McAlpine and A J Peacock; The pulmonary endothelium in health and disease, S Adnot *et al*; Pulmonary vascular control mechanisms in lung injury, N P Curzen *et al*; New perspectives in the treatment of pulmonary hypertension, A Y Butt and T W Higenbottam; Atrial natriuretic peptide and pulmonary hypertension, J S Thompson and A H Morice; The medical management of pulmonary hypertension, L J Rubin; Lung transplantation for pulmonary vascular disease, P A Corris; Heart-lung and lung transplantation for pulmonary hypertension, T Locke.

1 85578 074 7 Hardback   290 pages   £80.00/US$128.00   October 1995

Pulmonary Vascular Remodelling

J E Bishop and G J Laurent, *The Rayne Institute, London* and J T Reeves, *University of Colorado Health Sciences Center, Colorado, USA*

This book aims to promote a better understanding of the link between lung arterial structure and function, with the hope of ultimately improving the treatment of pulmonary hypertension.

Written by scientists and clinicians who specialize in pulmonary vascular research or medicine, it describes the changes that occur in the structure and function of the pulmonary vasculature during the development of pulmonary hypertension. Detailed information is given on the molecular and cellular mechanisms involved in this remodelling process.

1 85578 041 0 Hardback   288 pages   £80.00/US$128.00   June 1995

Portland Press, 59 Portland Place, London W1N 3AJ, UK
Tel: 0171 580 5530 Fax: 0171 323 1136 Email: sales@portlandpress.co.uk

Studies in Physiology Series

Neural Control of Skilled Human Movements

F W J Cody, *University of Manchester, UK*

Studies in Physiology No. 3

This textbook focuses on skilled movements in man, while drawing upon vital evidence obtained in other species. Attention is mainly directed at movements of the hand and arm, which have been studied most fully. The production of speech sounds is considered as another important example of skilled movement. Concise up-dates of current understanding of the roles of the main motor centres — cerebral cortex, basal ganglia, cerebellum and spinal cord — in skilled movement and its clinical impairments, are provided by neuroscientists renowned for their research expertise and enthusiasm for teaching.

Contents: Cortical control of skilled movements, R N Lemon; The basal ganglia, J C Rothwell; The posterior parietal cortex, the cerebellum and the visual guidance of movement, J Stein; Compensatory reflex mechanisms following limb displacements, V Dietz; The control of speech, D H McFarland and J P Lund; Impairment of skilled manipulation in patients with lesions of the motor system, K R Mills.

1 85578 081 X Paperback   120 pages   £19.95/US$32.00   December 1995

The Pathophysiology of the Gut and Airways: An Introduction

P L R Andrews and J G Widdicombe, *St George's Hospital Medical School, London, UK*

Studies in Physiology No. 1

This book examines the pathophysiological basis of a number of relatively common clinical problems of the gut and airways. These two systems share many similar physiological features which are reflected in the pathophysiological basis of the diseases and disorders reviewed.

Contents: Respiratory and gastro-intestinal parallels: real or contrived? G Burnstock; Non-adrenergic, non-cholinergic nerves in airways, P Barnes; Non-adrenergic, non-cholinergic motor systems in the gastro-intestinal tract, G Sanger; The pathophysiology of cystic fibrosis in the airways, D Geddes and E Alton; The pathophysiology of cystic fibrosis in the gastro-intestinal tract, J Hardcastle *et al*; Hypersecretion in the airways, N Mygind; Diarrhoea and intestinal hypersecretion, N Read; The pathophysiology of airway inflammation and mucosal damage in asthma, S Webber and D Corfield; The pathophysiology of gastric and duodenal ulcer, J Wallace *et al*; Coughing: An airway defensive reflex, G Sant'Ambrogio; Vomiting: A gastro-intestinal tract defensive reflex, P Andrews; Glossary; Index.

1 85578 022 4 Paperback   150 pages   £16.95/US$27.50   1993

Portland Press, 59 Portland Place, London W1N 3AJ, UK
Tel: 0171 580 5530   Fax: 0171 323 1136   Email: sales@portlandpress.co.uk

77666009 2